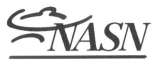

National
Association of
School Nurses

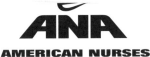

AMERICAN NURSES
ASSOCIATION

SCHOOL NURSING:
SCOPE AND STANDARDS
OF PRACTICE

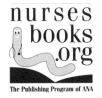

nurses
books
.org

The Publishing Program of ANA

AMERICAN NURSES ASSOCIATION
SILVER SPRING, MD
2005

Library of Congress Cataloging-in-Publication data

National Association of School Nurses (U.S.)
  School nursing : scope and standards of practice / National Association of School Nurses.
    p. ; cm.
  Includes bibliographical references and index.
  ISBN-13: 978-1-55810-227-9
  ISBN-10: 1-55810-227-2
  1. School nursing—Standards—United States.
  [DNLM: 1. School Nursing. 2. Nursing Process. WY 113 N277sh 2005] I. American Nurses Association. II. Title.

RJ247.N38 2005
371.7′12—dc22   2005014707

The American Nurses Association (ANA) is a national professional association. This ANA publication—*School Nursing: Scope and Standards of Practice*—reflects the thinking of the nursing profession on various issues and should be reviewed in conjunction with state board of nursing policies and practices. State law, rules, and regulations govern the practice of nursing, while *School Nursing: Scope and Standards of Practice* guides nurses in the application of their professional skills and responsibilities.

Published by Nursesbooks.org
The Publishing Program of ANA

American Nurses Association
8515 Georgia Avenue, Suite 400
Silver Spring, MD 20910
1-800-274-4ANA
http://www.nursingworld.org/

ANA is the only full-service professional organization representing the nation's 2.9 million Registered Nurses through its 54 constituent member associations. ANA advances the nursing profession by fostering high standards of nursing practice, promoting the economic and general welfare of nurses in the workplace, projecting a positive and realistic view of nursing, and lobbying the Congress and regulatory agencies on healthcare issues affecting nurses and the public.

The National Association of School Nurses is the leading worldwide expert for school health services and is the only organization that represents school nurses and school nursing interests exclusively. Its mission is to advance the delivery of professional school health services in order to promote optimal health and learning in students, primarily through its programs and resources for its members, advocacy and public relations activities, and research support and initiatives.

ISBN 13: 978-1-55810-227-9   SAN:851-3481   3M   07/08R

First Printing June 2005. Second Printing July 2006. Third Printing July 2007.
Fourth Printing July 2008.

CONTENTS

ACKNOWLEDGMENTS

The National Association of School Nurses wishes to acknowledge and thank the following organizational representatives who served on a task force to review the 2001 *Scope and Standards of Professional School Nursing Practice* and suggest revisions:

Roberta Bavin, MN, CPNP, CS
National Association of Pediatric Nurses and Practitioners

Julia Muennich Cowell, PhD, RNC, FAAN
American Public Health Association

Charlotte Burt, MSN, MA, RNBC, FASHA
American School Health Association

Linda Davis-Aldritt, RN, MA, PHN
National Association of State School Nurse Consultants

Maria Klein-Rivera, RNC, MSN
National Center for School Health Nursing

The National Association of School Nurses appreciates the work of the Board of Directors on this document and the following individuals for their expertise and contributions:

Carol Boal, BGS, RN, NCSN
NASN Executive Committee, Board of Directors, Wyoming

Sandi Delack, BSN, MEd, RN, CSNT
NASN Executive Committee, Board of Directors, Rhode Island

Cynthia Galemore, BSN, MSEd, RN, NCSN
NASN Executive Committee, Kansas

Janis Hootman, RN, PhD, NCSN
NASN President, Oregon

Sally Hrymak Hunter, RN, BSN, NCSN
NASN Vice President, New Mexico

Patricia Krin, MSN, APRN, FNP, NCSN
NASN Executive Committee, Connecticut

Wanda Miller, RN, MA, NCSN, FNASN
NASN Former President and Executive Director, Colorado

Norma Nikkola, RN, BS, MS
NASN Board, Ohio

Susan Praeger, RN, EdD
School Nurse Educator, Ohio

Susanne Tullos, RN, MNSc, MSBA, NCSN
NASN Secretary, Arkansas

Susan Will, RN, MPH, NCSN, FNASN
NASN President-elect, Minnesota

Linda C. Wolfe, RN, BSN, MEd, NCSN
NASN Past President, Delaware

In addition, I wish to thank Dr. Carol Bickford, Senior Policy Fellow of the Department of Nursing Practice and Policy of the American Nurses Association, for her many suggestions and unfailing support during the review and revision process.

Elizabeth L. Thomas, RN, BS, MEd, NCSN
NASN Task Force Leader and Editor, Delaware

ANA Staff

Carol J. Bickford, PhD, RN,BC – Content editor
Yvonne Humes, MSA – Project coordinator
Winifred Carson, JD – Legal counsel

PREFACE

The contents of this document have evolved over time to frame the current role and practice of school nurses in many locales across the country and in American schools abroad. School nursing has had standards of practice since 1983, when a task force of the National Association of School Nurses, chaired by Georgia McDonough of Arizona, produced the first set of standards specific to the specialty (ANA 1983). These were modeled on early generic standards authored by the American Nurses Association (ANA). The 1983 standards served school nursing well and were the basis for the development of three implementation manuals: one by the American School Health Association (Snyder 1991), and two by the National Association of School Nurses (Proctor 1990; Proctor, Lordi, and Zaiger 1993).

The scope of practice statement describes the who, what, where, when, why, and how of school nursing practice. Review and discussion by professional school nurses focused on answering these questions and resulted in the revised scope statement. Originally written by Leslie Cooper, RN, MSN, CS, FNP, and Donna Mazyck, RN, MS, NCSN, and first published with the standards in 2001, the Scope of Practice statement has been updated and expanded, but its character remains unchanged. The standards in this document are based on the template language in *Nursing: Scope and Standards of Practice* (ANA 2004). Careful additions and substitutions make this document unique to school nursing.

The scope and standards for school nursing were approved by the National Association of School Nurses Board of Directors in November 2004 and submitted to ANA's Committee on Nursing Practice Standards and Guidelines for review. In March 2005 the ANA Congress on Nursing Practice and Economics completed its review and approved the scope of practice statement for school nursing and acknowledged the standards of practice for school nursing.

Together, the scope statement and standards describe the professional expectations of school nurses. The standards serve as a definitive guide for role implementation, interpretation, and evaluation. They are useful for the writing of position descriptions for the school nurse and for planning relevant professional development programs. The scope and standards of school nursing practice are also used in conjunction with state nurse practice acts and other relevant laws or regulations to determine the adequacy of school nursing practice. This document further defines and clarifies the role of school nurses within schools and communities.

Dr. Janis Hootman, President of the National Association of School Nurses, often has spoken of the legacy that school nurses provide for their colleagues and clients. It is with great optimism that this framework is offered to school nurses to help them channel their vast energies into health and academic achievement for all students. The legacy of high expectations for a long healthy life and lifelong learning is a gift school nurses strive to give every day to their clients.

Introduction

The Standards of School Nursing Practice and their accompanying measurement criteria describe and measure a competent level of school nursing practice and professional performance. Built on ANA's *Nursing: Scope and Standards of Practice* (ANA 2004) for registered nurses, these standards are authoritative statements of the accountability, direction, and evaluation of individuals in this specialty nursing practice. Composed of two sets—the Standards of Practice and the Standards of Professional Performance—these standards define how outcomes for school nurse activities can be measured.

The Standards of Practice reflect the six steps of the nursing process (assessment, diagnosis, outcomes identification, implementation, planning, and evaluation), which is the foundation for the critical thinking of all registered nurses. The Standards of Professional Performance describe the expected behaviors expected of the nurse in the role of a school nurse.

Also included in this book is a detailed statement on the scope of school nursing practice. This discussion describes the context of this specialty practice, effectively answering the essential questions: the who, what, where, when, why, and how of school nursing practice.

Current nursing practice reflects a number of themes that underlie all nursing practice and have significant meaning for school nursing practice (ANA 2004):

- Providing age-appropriate and culturally and ethnically sensitive care
- Maintaining a safe environment
- Educating patients [clients] about healthy practices and treatment modalities
- Assuring continuity of care
- Coordinating the care across settings and among caregivers
- Managing information
- Communicating effectively
- Utilizing technology.

School nursing practice embraces and uses these themes in current practice. In fact, a communication standard was part of the *Scope and Standards of Professional School Nursing Practice* (NASN 2001). It is not a separate standard in the current publication because communication is part of each of the standards. Effective communication is still the cornerstone of the school nurse's practice.

Taken together, the contents of this book delineate the professional responsibilities of all school nurses engaged in clinical practice. This and other documents, such as position statements and issue briefs, could serve as the basis for:

- Quality improvement systems;
- Databases;
- Regulatory systems;
- Healthcare reimbursement and financial methodologies;
- Development and evaluation of nursing service delivery systems and organizational structures;
- Certification activities;
- Position descriptions and performance appraisals;
- Agency policies, procedures, and protocols; and
- Educational offerings.

Standards and practice guidelines must be evaluated regularly. School nurses are invited to provide feedback to the National Association of School Nurses regarding the usefulness, effectiveness, and comprehensiveness of this document. Keep in mind that it cannot account for all possible developments in practice. Guidelines, documents, and local protocols and procedures, as well as federal and state regulations and nurse practice acts, provide further direction.

STANDARDS OF SCHOOL NURSING PRACTICE:
STANDARDS OF PRACTICE

STANDARD 1. ASSESSMENT
The school nurse collects comprehensive data pertinent to the client's health or the situation.

STANDARD 2. DIAGNOSIS
The school nurse analyzes the assessment data to determine the diagnosis or issues.

STANDARD 3. OUTCOMES IDENTIFICATION
The school nurse identifies expected outcomes for a plan individualized to the client or the situation.

STANDARD 4. PLANNING
The school nurse develops a plan that prescribes strategies and alternatives to attain expected outcomes.

STANDARD 5. IMPLEMENTATION
The school nurse implements the identified plan.

STANDARD 5A: COORDINATION OF CARE
The school nurse coordinates care delivery.

STANDARD 5B: HEALTH TEACHING AND HEALTH PROMOTION
The school nurse provides health education and employs strategies to promote health and a safe environment.

STANDARD 5C: CONSULTATION
The school nurse provides consultation to influence the identified plan, enhance the abilities of others, and effect change.

STANDARD 5D: PRESCRIPTIVE AUTHORITY AND TREATMENT
The advanced practice registered nurse uses prescriptive authority, procedures, referrals, treatments, and therapies in accordance with state and federal laws and regulations.

STANDARD 6. EVALUATION
The school nurse evaluates progress towards achievement of outcomes.

Standards of School Nursing Practice: Standards of Professional Performance

Standard 7. Quality of Practice
The school nurse systematically enhances the quality and effectiveness of nursing practice.

Standard 8. Education
The school nurse attains knowledge and competency that reflects current school nursing practice.

Standard 9. Professional Practice Evaluation
The school nurse evaluates one's own nursing practice in relation to professional standards and guidelines, relevant statutes, rules, and regulations.

Standard 10. Collegiality
The school nurse interacts with, and contributes to the professional development of, peers and school personnel as colleagues.

Standard 11. Collaboration
The school nurse collaborates with the client, the family, school staff, and others in the conduct of school nursing practice.

Standard 12. Ethics
The school nurse integrates ethical provisions in all areas of practice.

Standard 13. Research
The school nurse integrates research findings into practice.

Standard 14. Resource Utilization
The school nurse considers factors related to safety, effectiveness, cost, and impact on practice in the planning and delivery of school nursing services.

Standard 15. Leadership
The school nurse provides leadership in the professional practice setting and the profession.

Standard 16. Program Management
The school nurse manages school health services.

SCOPE OF SCHOOL NURSING PRACTICE

Definitions and Distinguishing Characteristics

Nursing is the protection, promotion, and optimization of health and abilities, prevention of illness and injury, alleviation of suffering through the diagnosis and treatment of human response, and advocacy in the care of individuals, families, communities, and populations (ANA 2003a). "School Nursing is a specialized practice of professional nursing that advances the well-being, academic success, and lifelong achievement and health of students. To that end, school nurses facilitate positive student responses to normal development; promote health and safety; intervene with actual and potential health problems; provide case management services; and actively collaborate with others to build student and family capacity for adaptation, self-management, self advocacy, and learning" (NASN 1999b).

School nursing takes place primarily within local education agencies serving school-age children. However, school nurses also provide services in alternative sites (e.g., juvenile justice centers, alternative treatment centers, preschools, college campuses, learning sites for children of personnel in the armed services, and residential campuses) and within the larger surrounding community, at students' homes, vocational/occupational settings, environmental camps, field trips, school-sanctioned competitions, and sporting events.

The school nurse is likely to be the only healthcare provider in the educational setting. Unlike other healthcare workers—such as occupational therapists, physical therapists, and school psychologists, all of whom have specific defined caseloads—the school nurse is responsible for all students in a given school, district, or region. The school nurse collaborates with other health professionals to provide successful interventions for positive client outcomes. School nurses are frequently called upon to delegate nursing care to teachers, school office staff, classroom assistants, and other unlicensed assistive personnel (UAP). School nurses must be fully aware of the applicable laws, regulations, and standards pertaining to delegation of nursing tasks to others. Some states have laws or regulations prohibiting such delegation.

School nurses are most commonly employed by local school districts or education systems, although health systems such as public health, hospitals, and private health corporations may be the employer. School nurses work in a variety of delivery models such as consultant or direct services provider. They work with individuals, as well as populations, serving students from birth through age 21 or even older. The "client" of the school nurse includes not only the student, but also the student's family, the staff and faculty of the school, and the school community at large. Key roles of the school nurse include clinician, advocate, social service coordinator, health educator, liaison, and interdisciplinary student services team member (Wolfe 2005):

> Since the inception of school nursing, at the turn of the twentieth century, the specialty practice has embraced both health and education initiatives to promote the health and well-being of children. Lillian Wald, founder, envisioned a role for the school nurse to serve all, regardless of economic or social stature, or origin of nationality. She merged public health goals (to be free of communicable disease, which was of epidemic proportions), educational goals (to eliminate absenteeism from exclusion based upon contagious status), and social goals (to build literate and productive citizens). Medical goals focused on identification and exclusion of children. School nursing goals focused on inclusion.

In today's world, communicable diseases are not the only health related barriers to education. Some of the issues school nurses must address include:

- Child abuse and neglect;
- Domestic and school violence;
- Child and adolescent obesity and inactivity;
- Suicide;
- Alcohol, tobacco, and other drug use;
- Adolescent pregnancy and parenting;
- Environmental health;
- Physical and emotional disabilities and their consequences;
- Mental health;

- Children with complex physical needs; and
- Lack of health insurance coverage

School nursing is the pivotal component in continuity of care through the coordination, planning, delivery, and assessment of school health services. School nurses use the nursing process, the six steps of which—assessment, diagnosis, outcomes identification, implementation, planning, evaluation—and are the basis for the Standards of Practice. Among its other uses, this process helps to promote student and staff health and safety. School nurses also develop team relationships within the school and with community providers so that care is coordinated across settings to meet individual health needs and to avoid duplication of services.

The school nurse's primary role is to support student learning by acting as an advocate and liaison between the home, the school, and the medical community regarding concerns that may affect a student's ability to learn (NASN 1999b). Specific responsibilities are as diverse as the clients and communities served. The school nurse provides comprehensive services in all components of a coordinated school health program (Marx, Wooley, and Northrup 1998):

- Health services—Serves as the coordinator of the health services program, provides nursing care, advocates for health rights and optimization of health and abilities, and provides referral for services.

- Health education—Provides appropriate health information that promotes health and informed healthcare decisions, prevents disease, and enhances school performance.

- Environment—Identifies health and safety concerns in the school community, promotes a safe and nurturing school environment, and promotes injury prevention.

- Nutrition—Supports school food service programs and promotes the benefits of healthy eating patterns.

- Physical education and activity—Promotes healthy activities, physical education, and sports policies and practices that promote safety, good sportsmanship, and a lifelong active lifestyle.

- Counseling and mental health—Provides health counseling, assesses mental health needs, provides interventions, refers students to appropriate school staff or community agencies, and provides follow-up once treatment is prescribed.

- Parent and community involvement—Promotes community participation in assuring a healthy school and serves as school liaison to a health advisory committee.
- Staff wellness—Provides health education and counseling, and promotes healthy activities and environment for school staff.

Continuum of School Nursing Practice

School nursing exists on a continuum from the beginner through the veteran. Both the generalist school nurse and the school nurse practitioner with advanced practice training must hold current licensure as registered nurses in the state in which they practice.

Because of the complexity of issues addressed by the school nurse, the National Association of School Nurses (NASN) recommends as the minimum education for a school nurse a baccalaureate degree in nursing (BSN) from an accredited college or university, as well as state certification in states that require or recommend certification for state school nurses. Those school nurse generalists who have not acquired these credentials are strongly encouraged to aspire to and achieve these qualifications. NASN also recommends that school nurse generalists demonstrate their knowledge of school nursing by acquiring certification in the specialty of school nursing, which also requires a bachelor's degree. The NCSN credential is awarded by the National Board for Certification of School Nurses to those who pass the school nurse certification examination.

The continuum of school nurse practice includes other school nurse professionals such as advanced practice registered nurses, school nurse consultants, school nurse supervisors and administrators, lead nurses, or team leaders. There are school nurses in lead roles at school districts, regions, counties, and at the state level. As lifelong learners, school nurses seek professional development to increase critical thinking skills and professional judgment as well as to maintain current skills and knowledge. In some states, professional development is tied to licensure, but, in any case, school nurses have a professional responsibility to increase their own personal body of knowledge.

School nurses, whether generalists or advanced practice nurses, employ a community health focus in their practice. Health services are provided within the framework of primary, secondary, and tertiary pre-

vention. Programs and services are offered with the goal of prevention—to individual students as well as to the entire school community.

School Nurse

The school nurse provides health education, health promotion, preventive health services, health assessment, and referral services to clients
and staff. The actions of the school nurse focus on strengthening and
facilitating students' educational outcomes, and may be directed toward
individual students, family, segments of the school population, the entire
school population, the school community, or the larger surrounding
community. The school nurse serves as the liaison between the school,
community healthcare providers, and the school-based or school-linked
clinics. "As the healthcare expert within the school system, the school
nurse takes a leadership role in the development and evaluation of
school health policies. The school nurse participates in and provides
leadership to coordinated school health programs, crisis/disaster management teams, and school health advisory councils" (NASN 2002).

The school nurse must demonstrate expertise in pediatric and
adolescent health assessment, community health, and adult and child
mental health nursing. Strong skills in health promotion, assessment and
referral, communication, leadership, organization, and time management are essential. Knowledge of health and education laws that affect
students is critical, as are teaching strategies for the delivery of health
education to clients and staff, individually and collectively. School nurses
are often physically isolated from other nursing and healthcare colleagues; therefore they need to be comfortable and skilled with independent management of the health office and the client caseload
(Wolfe 2005).

The functions of the school nurse are to promote academic success
and provide optimal nursing care to the entire school community. To
these ends, the school nurse most often employs the six steps of the
nursing process (adapted from ANA 2004):

- Assessment—Collects comprehensive data.

- Diagnosis—Analyzes data to determine the *nursing* diagnoses or
  issues.

- Outcomes identification—Identifies *measurable* expected outcomes for a plan.

- Planning—Develops a plan to attain expected outcomes.
- Implementation—Implements the plan.
- Evaluation—Evaluates progress toward attainment of outcomes.

Advanced Practice Registered Nurse

Some school nurses may meet the standards for Advanced Practice Registered Nurses (APRNs) as a result of their education, experience, skill, and authority to practice by their state licensing board. APRNs have advanced degrees and national certification in their specialty. They can be nurse practitioners or clinical specialists or both. They are differentiated by educational preparation and clinical practice. APRNs are often part of an enhanced school services team that offers health care beyond basic core services. The APRN working in the school must be knowledgeable about and competent in the standards expected of the school nurse. APRNs can offer a cost-effective solution to identified needs for students who do not receive "consistent, appropriate medical care" contributing to barriers to learning. "The anticipated outcome is more health needs of students being met, resulting in a positive impact on the health and educational performance of students" (NASN 2003).

Nursing Role Specialty

Nursing role specialties are advanced levels of nursing practice that intersect with other bodies of knowledge, have a direct influence on nursing practice, and support the delivery of direct care rendered to patients by other registered nurses. School nurses with additional professional experience and education may elect to conduct their school nursing practice within administration, education, case management, informatics, research, or other role specialties. The school nurse in a nursing role specialty should have a master's or doctoral degree. The school nurse in a role specialty is expected to comply with the standards of practice and professional performance and the associated measurement criteria for all school nurses and the additional measurement criteria for the role specialist. Other resources, such as *Scope and Standards for Nurse Administrators* (ANA 2003b), may provide additional direction.

Ethical Considerations

The degree to which the school environment supports nursing practice affects the delivery of nursing care. *Healthy People 2010* cites a recommended school nurse to student ratio of 1:750 in the national health objectives (USDHHS 2000). The appropriateness of this ratio is dependent on the needs of the school population. School nurses must be able to practice nursing in an educationally focused system and clearly communicate in both the healthcare and education arenas. School nurses face unique policy, funding, and supervisory issues.

The school nurse practices in an environment that has changed dramatically since the early twentieth century. The Individuals with Disabilities Act of 1997, section 504 of the Rehabilitation Act of 1973, and the Americans with Disabilities Act of 1990 removed barriers that hindered students' access to education. Education regulations heighten the complexity of decision-making and practice, such as those of the Family Education Rights and Privacy Act (FERPA) of 1974, and subsequent amendments regarding Do Not Resuscitate orders in the school setting. The restrictions to medical information imposed by the Health Information Portability and Accessibility Act (HIPAA) of 1996 present an ongoing challenge to the school nurse who needs information about student medical needs for adequate care at school.

School nurses are advocates for their clients—students, families, school staff, and the community. They provide care to their clients that is both age-appropriate and culturally and ethnically sensitive. School nurses promote active informed participation in health decisions. They respect the individual's right to be treated with dignity, and understand the ethical and legal issues surrounding an individual's right to privacy and confidentiality. The school nurse treats all members of the school community equally, regardless of race, gender, social or economic status, culture, age, sexual orientation, disability, or religion.

The school nurse maintains the highest level of competency by enhancing professional knowledge and skills, collaborating with peers and other health professionals and community agencies, and adhering to these documents: *Nursing's Social Policy Statement* (ANA 2003a), *Code of Ethics for Nurses with Interpretive Statements* (ANA 2001), *Code of Ethics with Interpretive Statements for the School Nurse* (NASN 1999a), and the current scope and standards of school nursing. School nurses participate in the profession's efforts to advance the standards of practice, expand the body of knowledge through nursing research, and improve conditions of employment. School nurses are expected to regulate themselves; they are responsible to themselves and others for the quality of their practice. The school nurse is autonomous and must engage in considerable reflection for quality assurance.

Summary

School nurses continue to adapt their practice to a changing world. New challenges continue to present themselves, as do new tools to assist the school nurse in meeting these challenges. As technology advances, so does the school nurse's practice. Students with more complex daily health needs, as well as those requiring intermittent on-site medical treatments, are in schools across America every day. Technology is available, not only as a classroom tool and for expanded school health record keeping, but also to give students with health impairments greater access to the education to which they are entitled.

Healthy children are successful learners. The school nurse has a multifaceted role within the school setting, one that supports the physical, emotional, mental, and social health of students and their success in the learning process (NASN 2002). The future of school nursing rests on the ability of the school nurse to successfully meet the challenges in the health and education communities.

Standards of School Nursing Practice
Standards of Practice

> *School Nursing is a specialized practice of professional nursing that advances the well-being, academic success, and lifelong achievement and health of students. To that end, school nurses facilitate positive student responses to normal development; promote health and safety; intervene with actual and potential health problems; provide case management services; and actively collaborate with others to build student and family capacity for adaptation, self-management, self-advocacy, and learning.* (NASN 1999b)

Standard 1. Assessment
The school nurse collects comprehensive data pertinent to the client's* health or the situation.

Measurement Criteria:

The school nurse:

- Systematically compares and contrasts clinical findings with normal and abnormal variations and developmental events in forming a nursing diagnosis.

- Involves the client, family, school staff, other healthcare providers, and school community, as appropriate, in holistic data collection.

- Prioritizes data collection activities based on the client's immediate condition, or anticipated needs of the client or situation.

- Uses appropriate evidence-based assessment techniques and instruments in collecting pertinent data.

- Uses analytical models and problem-solving tools.

---

* *Client* is used in these standards to better reflect the diversity of the recipients of school nursing practice. The client can be a student, the student and family as a unit, the school population, or the school community, including faculty and staff. The focus of care may shift from individual needs to the needs of a group.

Continued ▶

- Synthesizes available data, information, and knowledge relevant to the situation to identify patterns and variances.
- Documents relevant data in a retrievable format.

Additional Measurement Criterion for the Advanced Practice Registered Nurse:
The advanced practice registered nurse:

- Initiates and interprets diagnostic tests and procedures relevant to the client's current status.

STANDARD 2. DIAGNOSIS
The school nurse analyzes the assessment data to determine the diagnoses or issues.

Measurement Criteria:

The school nurse:

- Derives the nursing diagnoses or issues based on assessment data.

- Validates the nursing diagnoses or issues with the client, family, school staff, school community, and other healthcare providers when possible and appropriate.

- Documents nursing diagnoses or issues in a manner that facilitates the determination of the expected outcomes and plan.

- Uses standardized language or recognized terminology to document the nursing diagnosis in a retrievable form.

Additional Measurement Criteria for the Advanced Practice Registered Nurse:

The advanced practice registered nurse:

- Systematically compares and contrasts clinical findings with normal and abnormal variations and developmental events in formulating a differential diagnosis.

- Utilizes complex data and information obtained during interview, examination, and diagnostic procedures in identifying diagnoses.

- Assists staff in developing and maintaining competency in the diagnostic process.

STANDARD 3. OUTCOMES IDENTIFICATION
The school nurse identifies expected outcomes for a plan individualized to the client or the situation.

Measurement Criteria:

The school nurse:

- Involves the client, family, school staff, and other healthcare providers in formulating expected outcomes when possible and appropriate.
- Derives culturally appropriate expected outcomes from the diagnoses.
- Considers associated risks, benefits, costs, current scientific evidence, and clinical expertise when formulating expected outcomes.
- Defines expected outcomes in terms of the client, client values, ethical considerations, environment, or situation with such consideration as associated risks, benefits and costs, and current scientific evidence.
- Includes a time estimate for attainment of expected outcomes.
- Develops expected outcomes that provide direction for continuity of care.
- Modifies expected outcomes based on changes in the status of the client or evaluation of the situation.
- Documents expected outcomes as measurable goals.
- Uses standardized language or recognized terminology to document the outcome in a retrievable form.

Additional Measurement Criteria for the Advanced Practice Registered Nurse:

The advanced practice registered nurse:

- Identifies expected outcomes that incorporate scientific evidence and are achievable through implementation of evidence-based practices.

- Identifies expected outcomes that incorporate cost and clinical effectiveness, client satisfaction, and continuity and consistency among providers.

- Supports the use of clinical guidelines linked to positive client outcomes.

STANDARD 4. PLANNING
The school nurse develops a plan that prescribes strategies and alternatives to attain expected outcomes.

Measurement Criteria:

The school nurse:

- Develops an individualized healthcare plan considering the client characteristics or the situation (e.g., age and culturally appropriate, environmentally sensitive), with appropriate strategies for health promotion and disease prevention.

- Develops the plan in conjunction with the client, family, school community, and others, as appropriate.

- Creates individual healthcare plans as a component of the program for clients with special healthcare needs.

- Provides for continuity within the plan.

- Incorporates an implementation pathway or timeline within the plan.

- Establishes the plan priorities with the client, family, school community, and others as appropriate.

- Utilizes the plan to provide direction to other members of the school team.

- Defines the plan to reflect current statutes, rules and regulations, and standards.

- Integrates current trends and research affecting care in the planning process.

- Considers the economic impact of the plan.

- Uses standardized language or recognized terminology to document the plan in a retrievable form.

Additional Measurement Criteria for the Advanced Practice Registered Nurse:

The advanced practice registered nurse:

- Identifies assessment, diagnostic strategies, and therapeutic interventions within the plan that reflect current evidence, including data, research, literature, and expert clinical knowledge.

- Selects or designs strategies to meet the multifaceted needs of complex clients.
- Includes the synthesis of client's values and beliefs regarding nursing and medical therapies within the plan.

Additional Measurement Criteria for the Nursing Role Specialty:

The school nurse in a nursing role specialty:

- Participates in the design and development of multidisciplinary and interdisciplinary processes to address the situation or issue.
- Contributes to the development and continuous improvement of organizational systems that support the planning process.
- Supports the integration of clinical, human, and financial resources to enhance and complete the decision-making processes.

Standard 5. Implementation
The school nurse implements the identified plan.

Measurement Criteria:

The school nurse:

- Implements the plan in a safe and timely manner.
- Documents implementation and any modifications, including changes or omissions, of the specified plan.
- Utilizes evidence-based interventions and treatments specific to the diagnosis or problem.
- Utilizes community resources and systems to implement the plan.
- Collaborates with nursing colleagues and others to implement the plan.
- Provides interventions in compliance with these standards of practice and professional performance.
- Uses standardized language or recognized terminology to document implementation of the plan in a retrievable form.

Additional Measurement Criteria for the Advanced Practice Registered Nurse:

The advanced practice registered nurse:

- Facilitates utilization of systems and community resources to implement the plan.
- Supports collaboration with school nursing colleagues and other nursing colleagues and disciplines to implement the plan.
- Incorporates new knowledge and strategies to initiate change in school nursing care practices if desired outcomes are not achieved.

Additional Measurement Criteria for the Nursing Role Specialty:

The school nurse in a nursing role specialty:

- Implements the plan using principles and concepts of project or systems management.
- Fosters organizational systems that support implementation of the plan.

STANDARD 5A: COORDINATION OF CARE
The school nurse coordinates care delivery.

Measurement Criteria:

The school nurse:

- Coordinates creation and implementation of the individual health-care plan.
- Documents the coordination of the care.

Measurement Criteria for the Advanced Practice Registered Nurse:

The advanced practice registered nurse:

- Provides leadership in the coordination of multidisciplinary health care for integrated delivery of client care services.
- Synthesizes data and information to prescribe necessary education and healthcare system and community support measures, including environmental modifications.
- Coordinates education and healthcare system and community resources that enhance delivery of care across continuums.

STANDARD 5B: HEALTH TEACHING AND HEALTH PROMOTION
The school nurse provides health education and employs strategies to promote health and a safe environment.

Measurement Criteria:

The school nurse:

- Provides general health education to the student body at large through direct classroom instruction or expert consultation.

- Provides health teaching that addresses such topics as healthy lifestyles, risk-reducing behaviors, developmental needs, activities of daily living, and preventive self-care as appropriate to client developmental levels.

- Uses health promotion and health teaching methods appropriate to the situation and the client's developmental level, learning needs, readiness, ability to learn, language preference, and culture.

- Promotes self-care and safety through the education of the school community regarding health issues.*

- Promotes health principles through the coordinated school health program for all in the school community.

- Seeks opportunities for feedback and evaluation of the effectiveness of the strategies used.

- Participates in the assessment of needs for health education and health instruction for the school community.*

- Provides individual and group health teaching and counseling for and with clients.*

- Participates in the design and development of health education materials, and other health education activities.*

- Participates in the evaluation of health curricula and health instructional materials and activities.*

- Acts as a primary resource person to school staff (and others as appropriate) regarding health education and health education materials.*

---

*Adapted from Proctor, Lordi, and Zaiger 1993 and NASN and ANA 2001.

Additional Measurement Criteria for the Advanced Practice Registered Nurse:

The advanced practice registered nurse:

- Synthesizes empirical evidence on risk behaviors, learning theories, behavioral change theories, motivational theories, epidemiology, and other related theories and frameworks when designing health information and client education.

- Designs health information and client education appropriate to the client's developmental level, learning needs, readiness to learn, and cultural values and beliefs.

- Evaluates health information resources, such as the Internet, within the area of practice for accuracy, readability, and comprehensibility to help client's access quality health information.

Standard 5c: Consultation
The school nurse provides consultation to influence the identified plan, enhance the abilities of others, and effect change.

Measurement Criteria:

The school nurse:

- Synthesizes data, information, theoretical frameworks, and evidence when providing consultation.

- Facilitates the effectiveness of a consultation by involving the stakeholders in the decision-making process.

- Communicates consultation recommendations that influence the identified plan, facilitate understanding by involved stakeholders, enhance the work of others, and effect change.

Measurement Criteria for the Advanced Practice Registered Nurse:

The advanced practice registered nurse:

- Synthesizes clinical data, theoretical frameworks, and evidence when providing consultation.

- Facilitates the effectiveness of a consultation by involving the client when appropriate in decision-making and negotiating role responsibilities.

- Communicates consultation recommendations that facilitate change.

STANDARD 5D: PRESCRIPTIVE AUTHORITY AND TREATMENT
The advanced practice registered nurse uses prescriptive authority, procedures, referrals, treatments, and therapies in accordance with state and federal laws and regulations.

Measurement Criteria for the Advanced Practice Registered Nurse:

The advanced practice registered nurse:

- Prescribes evidence-based treatments, therapies, and procedures considering the client's comprehensive healthcare needs.

- Prescribes pharmacologic agents based on a current knowledge of pharmacology and physiology.

- Prescribes specific pharmacological agents and/or treatments based on clinical indicators, the client's status and needs, and the results of diagnostic and laboratory tests.

- Evaluates therapeutic and potential adverse effects of pharmacological and non-pharmacological treatments.

- Provides client and family with information about intended effects and potential adverse effects of proposed prescriptive therapies.

- Provides information about costs, and alternative treatments and procedures, as appropriate.

STANDARD 6. EVALUATION
The school nurse evaluates progress towards attainment of outcomes.

Measurement Criteria:

The school nurse:

- Conducts a systematic, ongoing, and criterion-based evaluation of the outcomes in relation to the structures and processes prescribed by the plan and the indicated timeline.

- Includes the client and others involved in the care or situation in the evaluative process.

- Evaluates the effectiveness of the planned strategies in relation to client responses and the attainment of the expected outcomes.

- Documents the results of the evaluation.

- Uses ongoing assessment data to revise the diagnoses, the outcomes, the plan, and the implementation as needed.

- Disseminates the results to the client and others involved in the care or situation, as appropriate, in accordance with client and parent directions, and state and federal laws and regulations.

Additional Measurement Criteria for the Advanced Practice Registered Nurse:

The advanced practice registered nurse:

- Evaluates the accuracy of the diagnosis and effectiveness of the interventions in relationship to the patient's attainment of expected outcomes.

- Synthesizes the results of the evaluation analyses to determine the impact of the plan on the affected clients, families, groups, communities, and institutions.

- Uses the results of the evaluation analyses to make or recommend process or structural changes, including policy, procedure, or protocol documentation, as appropriate.

Additional Measurement Criteria for the Nursing Role Specialty:

The school nurse in a nursing role specialty:

- Uses the results of the evaluation analyses to make or recommend process or structural changes, including policy, procedure, or protocol documentation, as appropriate.

- Synthesizes the results of the evaluation analyses to determine the impact of the plan on the affected clients, families, groups, school communities, and institutions, networks, and organizations.

Standards of Professional Performance

Standard 7. Quality of Practice
The school nurse systematically enhances the quality and effectiveness of nursing practice.

Measurement Criteria:

The school nurse:

- Demonstrates quality by documenting the application of the nursing process in a responsible, accountable, and ethical manner.

- Uses the results of quality improvement activities to initiate changes in school nursing practice and in the healthcare delivery system.

- Uses creativity and innovation in school nursing practice to improve care delivery.

- Incorporates new knowledge to initiate changes in school nursing practice if desired outcomes are not achieved.

- Participates in quality improvement activities. Such activities may include:

  - Identifying aspects of practice important for quality monitoring.

  - Using indicators developed to monitor quality and effectiveness of nursing practice.

  - Collecting data to monitor quality and effectiveness of school nursing practice.

  - Analyzing quality data to identify opportunities for improving school nursing practice.

  - Formulating recommendations to improve school nursing practice or outcomes.

  - Implementing activities to enhance the quality of school nursing practice.

Continued ▶

- Developing, implementing, and evaluating policies, procedures and/or guidelines to improve the quality of school nursing practice.

- Participating on interdisciplinary teams to evaluate clinical care or health services.

- Participating in efforts to minimize costs and unnecessary duplication.

- Analyzing factors related to safety, satisfaction, effectiveness, and cost–benefit options.

- Analyzing organizational systems for barriers.

- Obtaining and maintaining national certification in school nursing as well as state certification (if available).

- Implementing processes to remove or decrease barriers within organizational systems.

Additional Measurement Criteria for the Advanced Practice Registered Nurse:

The advanced practice registered nurse:

- Obtains and maintains professional certification if available in the area of expertise.

- Designs quality improvement initiatives.

- Implements initiatives to evaluate the need for change.

- Evaluates the practice environment and quality of nursing care rendered in relation to existing evidence, identifying opportunities for the generation and use of research.

Additional Measurement Criteria for the Nursing Role Specialty:

The school nurse in a nursing role specialty:

- Obtains and maintains professional certification if available in the area of expertise.

- Designs quality improvement initiatives.

- Implements initiatives to evaluate the need for change.

- Evaluates the practice environment in relation to existing evidence, identifying opportunities for the generation and use of research.

STANDARD 8. EDUCATION
The school nurse attains knowledge and competency that reflects current school nursing practice.

Measurement Criteria:

The school nurse:

- Participates in ongoing educational activities related to appropriate knowledge bases and professional issues.

- Demonstrates a commitment to lifelong learning through self-reflection and inquiry to identify learning needs.

- Seeks experiences that reflect current practice in order to maintain skills and competence in clinical practice or role performance.

- Acquires knowledge and skills appropriate to the specialty area, practice setting, role, or situation.

- Maintains professional records that provide evidence of competency and lifelong learning.

- Seeks experiences and formal and independent learning activities to maintain and develop clinical and professional skills and knowledge.

Additional Measurement Criterion for the Advanced Practice Registered Nurse:

The advanced practice registered nurse:

- Uses current healthcare research findings and other evidence to expand clinical knowledge, enhance role performance, and increase knowledge of professional issues.

Additional Measurement Criterion for the Nursing Role Specialty:

The school nurse in a nursing role specialty:

- Uses current research findings and other evidence to expand knowledge, enhance role performance, and increase knowledge of professional issues.

STANDARD 9. PROFESSIONAL PRACTICE EVALUATION

The school nurse evaluates one's own nursing practice in relation to professional practice standards and guidelines, relevant statutes, rules, and regulations.

Measurement Criteria:

- The school nurse's practice reflects the application of knowledge of current practice standards, guidelines, statutes, rules, and regulations.

- The school nurse:

  - Provides age-appropriate care in a culturally and ethnically sensitive manner.

  - Engages in self-evaluation of practice on a regular basis, identifying areas of strength as well as areas in which professional development would be beneficial.

  - Obtains informal feedback regarding one's own practice from clients, peers, professional colleagues, and others.

  - Participates in systematic peer review as appropriate.

  - Takes action to achieve goals identified during the evaluation process.

  - Provides rationales for practice beliefs, decisions, and actions as part of the informal and formal evaluation processes.

Additional Measurement Criterion for the Advanced Practice Registered Nurse:

The advanced practice registered nurse:

- Engages in a formal process seeking feedback regarding one's own practice from clients, peers, professional colleagues, and others.

Additional Measurement Criterion for the Nursing Role Specialty:

The school nurse in a nursing role specialty:

- Engages in a formal process seeking feedback regarding role performance from individuals, professional colleagues, representatives and administrators of corporate entities, and others.

STANDARD 10. COLLEGIALITY

The school nurse interacts with, and contributes to the professional development of, peers and school personnel as colleagues.

Measurement Criteria:

The school nurse:

- Shares knowledge and skills with peers and colleagues as evidenced by such activities as multidisciplinary student assistance conferences or presentations at formal or informal meetings.

- Provides peers with feedback regarding their practice or role performance.

- Interacts with peers and colleagues to enhance one's own professional nursing practice and role performance and the health care of the school community.

- Maintains compassionate and caring relationships with peers and colleagues.

- Contributes to an environment that is conducive to the education of healthcare professionals and the whole school community.

- Contributes to a supportive and healthy work environment.

- Participates in appropriate professional organizations in a membership or leadership capacity.

Additional Measurement Criteria for the Advanced Practice Registered Nurse:

The advanced practice registered nurse:

- Models expert practice to interdisciplinary team members and healthcare consumers.

- Mentors other registered nurses and colleagues as appropriate.

- Participates with interdisciplinary teams that contribute to role development and advanced nursing practice and health care.

Continued ▶

Additional Measurement Criteria for the Nursing Role Specialty:

The school nurse in a nursing role specialty:

- Participates on multi-professional teams that contribute to role development and, directly or indirectly, advance nursing practice and health services.

- Mentors other registered nurses and colleagues as appropriate.

STANDARD 11. COLLABORATION
The school nurse collaborates with the client, the family, school staff, and others in the conduct of school nursing practice.

Measurement Criteria:

The school nurse:

- Communicates with the client, the family, and healthcare providers regarding client care and the school nurse's role in the delivery of that care.

- Collaborates in creating a documented healthcare plan that is focused on outcomes and decisions related to care and delivery of services and indicates communication with clients, families, and others.

- Partners with others to effect change and generate positive outcomes through knowledge of the client or situation.

- Documents referrals, including provisions for continuity of care.

Additional Measurement Criteria for the Advanced Practice Registered Nurse:

The advanced practice registered nurse:

- Partners with other disciplines to enhance patient care through interdisciplinary activities, such as education, consultation, management, technological development, or research opportunities.

- Facilitates an interdisciplinary process with other members of the healthcare team.

- Documents plan-of-care communications, rationales for plan-of-care changes, and collaborative discussions to improve patient care.

Additional Measurement Criteria for the Nursing Role Specialty:

The school nurse in a nursing role specialty:

- Partners with others to enhance health care, and ultimately client care, through interdisciplinary activities such as education, consultation, management, technological development, or research.

- Documents plans, communications, rationales for plan changes, and collaborative discussions.

STANDARD 12. ETHICS
The school nurse integrates ethical provisions in all areas of practice.

Measurement Criteria:

The school nurse:

- Uses *Code of Ethics for Nurses with Interpretive Statements* (ANA 2001) and *Code of Ethics with Interpretive Statements for School Nurses* (NASN 1999a) to guide practice.

- Delivers care in a manner that preserves and protects client autonomy, dignity, and rights, sensitive to diversity in the school setting.

- Maintains client confidentiality within legal and regulatory parameters of both health and education.

- Serves as a client advocate assisting clients in developing skills for self-advocacy.

- Maintains a therapeutic and professional client–nurse relationship with appropriate professional role boundaries.

- Demonstrates a commitment to practicing self-care, managing stress, and connecting with self and others.

- Contributes to resolving ethical issues of clients, colleagues, or systems as evidenced in such activities as participating on ethics committees.

- Reports illegal, incompetent, or impaired practices.

- Seeks available resources to formulate ethical decisions.

Additional Measurement Criteria for the Advanced Practice Registered Nurse:

The advanced practice registered nurse:

- Informs the client of the risks, benefits, and outcomes of healthcare regimens.

- Participates in interdisciplinary teams that address ethical risks, benefits, and outcomes.

Additional Measurement Criteria for the Nursing Role Specialty:

The school nurse in a nursing role specialty:

- Participates on multidisciplinary and interdisciplinary teams that address ethical risks, benefits, and outcomes.

- Informs administrators or others of the risks, benefits, and outcomes of programs and decisions that affect healthcare delivery.

STANDARD 13. RESEARCH
The school nurse integrates research findings into practice.

Measurement Criteria:

The school nurse:

- Utilizes the best available evidence, including research findings, to guide practice decisions.
- Actively participates in research activities at various levels appropriate to the school nurse's education and position. Such activities may include:
    - Identifying clinical problems specific to nursing research (client care and nursing practice).
    - Participating in data collection (surveys, pilot projects, formal studies).
    - Participating in a formal committee or program.
    - Sharing research activities or findings with peers and others.
    - Conducting research.
    - Critically analyzing and interpreting research for application to practice.
    - Using research findings in the development of policies, procedures, and standards of practice in client care.
    - Incorporating research as a basis for learning.
    - Contributing to school nursing literature.

Additional Measurement Criteria for the Advanced Practice Registered Nurse:

The advanced practice registered nurse:

- Contributes to nursing knowledge by conducting or synthesizing research that discovers, examines, and evaluates knowledge, theories, criteria, and creative approaches to improve healthcare practice.
- Formally disseminates research findings through activities such as presentations, publications, consultation, and journal clubs.

Additional Measurement Criteria for the Nursing Role Specialty:

The school nurse in a nursing role specialty:

- Contributes to nursing knowledge by conducting or synthesizing research that discovers, examines, and evaluates knowledge, theories, criteria, and creative approaches to improve health care.

- Formally disseminates research findings through activities such as presentations, publications, consultation, and journal clubs.

STANDARD 14. RESOURCE UTILIZATION

The school nurse considers factors related to safety, effectiveness, cost, and impact on practice in the planning and delivery of school nursing services.

Measurement Criteria:

The school nurse:

- Evaluates factors such as safety, effectiveness, availability, cost and benefits, efficiencies, and impact on practice, when choosing among practice options that would result in the same expected outcome.

- Assists the client and family in identifying and securing appropriate and available services to address health-related needs.

- Assigns or delegates tasks, based on the needs and condition of the client, potential for harm, stability of the client's condition, complexity of the task, and predictability of the outcome; as defined and permitted by individual state nurse practice acts; and according to the knowledge and skills of the designated caregiver.

- Assists the client and school community in becoming informed consumers about the options, costs, risks, and benefits of health promotion, health education, school health services, and individualized health interventions for clients.

Additional Measurement Criteria for the Advanced Practice Registered Nurse:

The advanced practice registered nurse:

- Utilizes organizational and community resources to formulate multidisciplinary or interdisciplinary plans of care.

- Develops innovative solutions for client care problems that address effective resource utilization and maintenance of quality.

- Develops evaluation strategies to demonstrate cost effectiveness, cost–benefit, and efficiency factors associated with nursing practice.

Additional Measurement Criteria for the Nursing Role Specialty:

The school nurse in a nursing role specialty:

- Develops innovative solutions and applies strategies to obtain appropriate resources for nursing initiatives.

- Secures organizational resources to ensure a work environment conducive to completing the identified plan and outcomes.

- Develops evaluation methods to measure safety and effectiveness for interventions and outcomes.

- Promotes activities that assist others, as appropriate, in becoming informed about costs, risks, and benefits of care or of the plan and solution.

STANDARD 15. LEADERSHIP
The school nurse provides leadership in the professional practice setting and the profession.

Measurement Criteria:

The school nurse:

- Engages in teamwork as a team player and a team builder.

- Works to create and maintain healthy work environments in local, regional, national, or international communities.

- Displays the ability to define a clear vision, the associated goals, and a plan to implement and measure progress

- Demonstrates a commitment to continuous, lifelong learning for self and others.

- Teaches others to succeed by mentoring and other strategies.

- Exhibits creativity and flexibility through times of change.

- Demonstrates energy, excitement, and a passion for quality work.

- Willingly accepts mistakes by self and others, thereby creating a culture in which risk-taking is not only safe, but also expected.

- Inspires loyalty by valuing people as the most precious asset in an organization.

- Directs the coordination of care across settings and among caregivers, including oversight of licensed and unlicensed personnel in any assigned or delegated tasks as permitted by state nurse practice acts.

- Serves in key roles in the school and work settings by participating on committees, councils, and administrative teams.

- Promotes advancement of the profession through participation in professional school nursing and school health organizations.

- Demonstrates knowledge of the philosophy and mission of the school district, the nature of its curricular and extracurricular activities, and its programs and special services.*

---

*Adapted from Proctor, Lordi, and Zaiger 1993.

- Demonstrates knowledge of the roles of other school profession-als and adjunct personnel.*
- Coordinates roles and responsibilities of the adjunct school health personnel within the school team.*

Additional Measurement Criteria for the Advanced Practice Registered Nurse:

The advanced practice registered nurse:

- Works to influence decision-making bodies to improve client care.
- Provides direction to enhance the effectiveness of the healthcare team.
- Initiates and revises protocols or guidelines to reflect evidence-based practice, to reflect accepted changes in care management, or to address emerging problems.
- Promotes communication of information and advancement of the profession through writing, publishing, and presentations for pro-fessional or lay audiences.
- Designs innovations to effect change in practice and improve health outcomes.

Additional Measurement Criteria for the Nursing Role Specialty:

The school nurse in a nursing role specialty:

- Works to influence decision-making bodies to improve client care, health services, and policies.
- Promotes communication of information and advancement of the profession through writing, publishing, and presentations for pro-fessional or lay audiences.
- Designs innovations to effect change in practice and outcomes.
- Provides direction to enhance the effectiveness of the multi-disciplinary or interdisciplinary team.

STANDARD 16. PROGRAM MANAGEMENT
The school nurse manages school health services.

Measurement Criteria:

The school nurse:

- Manages school health services as appropriate to the nurse's education, position, and practice environment.*

- Conducts school health needs assessments to identify current health problems and identify the need for new programs.*

- Develops and implements needed health programs using a program planning process.*

- Demonstrates knowledge of existing school health programs and current health trends that may affect client care, the sources of funds for each, school policy related to each, and local, state, and federal laws governing each.*

- Develops and implements health policies and procedures in collaboration with the school administration, the board of health, and the board of education.*

- Evaluates ongoing health programs for outcomes and quality of care, and communicates findings to administrators and the board of education.*

- Orients, trains, documents competency, supervises, and evaluates health assistants, aides, and UAPs (unlicensed assistive personnel), as appropriate to the school setting.*

- Initiates changes throughout the healthcare delivery system, as appropriate, using the results of school health environmental needs assessments, analysis of evaluation data, and quality-of-care activities.*

- Participates in environmental safety and health activities (e.g., indoor air quality, injury surveillance and prevention).*

- Adopts and uses available technology appropriate to the work setting.*

---

*Adapted from Proctor, Lordi, and Zaiger 1993.

GLOSSARY

Client. Recipient of (school) nursing practice (ANA 2004). The client can be a student, the student and family as a unit, the school population, or the school community (faculty and staff). The focus of care may shift from individual needs to the needs of a group.

Plan. A comprehensive outline of components of care to be delivered to attain expected outcomes (ANA 2004). This would include an individualized healthcare plan (IHP), an individualized education plan (IEP) as part of the special education regulations (IDEA), a 504 plan, and others.

Role specialty. A practice in which the school nurse primarily works in education, case management, health education, prevention (such as adolescent pregnancy and parenting, or infectious disease), program implementation (such as special education or 504 plan creation and implementation), disease specialization (such as diabetes, asthma, or cystic fibrosis), administration, or leadership (such as lead nurse or co-ordinator for a large school district). This practice requires advanced study at the master's or doctoral level and considerable expertise.

School community. All those who study and work in a school district. This could be expanded when appropriate to community agencies, faith-based groups, student families, and others.

REFERENCES

American Nurses Association (ANA). 1983. Standards for professional nursing education. Kansas City, MO: ANA.

———. 2001. *Code of ethics for nurses with interpretive statements.* Washington, DC: American Nurses Publishing.

———. 2003. *Nursing's social policy statement.* 2nd Edition. Washington, DC: Nursebooks.org.

———. 2003. *Scope and standards for nurse administrators.* 2nd Edition. Washington, DC: Nursebooks.org.

———. 2004. *Nursing: Scope and standards of practice.* Washington, DC: Nursebooks.org.

Marx, E., S. Wooley, and D. Northrup, eds. 1998. *Health is academic: A guide to coordinated school health programs.* New York: Teacher's College Press.

National Association of School Nurses (NASN). 1999a. *Code of ethics with interpretive statements for school nurses.* Scarborough, ME: NASN.

———. 1999b. Definition of school nursing. Adopted at Board of Directors Meeting, June, Providence, RI.

——— and American Nurses Association (ANA). 2001. *Scope and standards of professional school nursing practice.* Washington, DC: American Nurses Publishing.

———. 2002. *Issue brief: School health nursing services role in health care.* Scarborough, ME: NASN.

———. 2003. *Position statement: Role of advanced nurse practitioner in the school setting.* Scarborough, ME: NASN.

Proctor, S.T. 1990. *Guidelines for a model school nurse services program.* Scarborough, ME: NASN.

Proctor, S.T., S.L. Lordi, and D.S. Zaiger. 1993. *School nursing practice: Roles and standards.* Scarborough, ME: NASN.

Synder, A. (ed.). 1991. *Implementation guide for the standards of school nursing practice.* Kent, OH: American School Health Association.

U.S. Department of Health and Human Services (USDHHS). 2000. *Healthy people 2010: Health objectives for the nation.* Washington, DC: USDHHS.

Wolfe, L. 2005. Roles of the school nurse. In *School nursing: A comprehensive text,* ed. J. Selekman. Philadelphia: F.A. Davis.

APPENDIX A
SCOPE AND STANDARDS OF
PROFESSIONAL SCHOOL NURSING PRACTICE (2001)

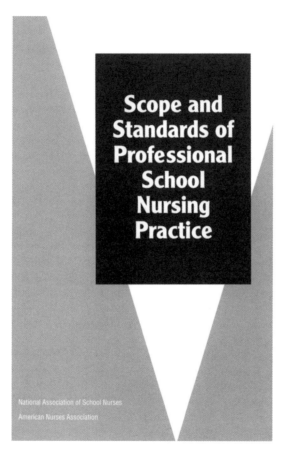

CONTENTS

PREFACE

The contents of this document are the result of an effort by a group of nurses comprised of representatives of several organizations concerned with the practice of nursing in schools.

The National Association of School Nurses Standards of Practice Task Force was charged with the development of new national standards of practice for school nursing. In particular, the new standards were to reflect the format and language of the *Standards of Clinical Nursing Practice 2nd Edition* (ANA 1998), a publication that specifies areas of responsibility and accountability common to the practice of all professional nurses. Formulated by the Committee on Nursing Practice Standards and Guidelines of the American Nurses Association, the *Standards of Clinical Nursing Practice 2nd Edition* establish criteria for all of nursing practice and serve as a template for the development of specialty standards.

School nursing has had standards of practice since 1983 when a similar task force, chaired by Georgia MacDonough of Arizona, produced the first set of standards specific to the specialty (ANA 1983). Similarly, these were modeled on early generic (non-specialty) standards also authored by the American Nurses Association. The 1983 standards served school nursing well and were the basis for the development of three implementation manuals: one by the American School Health Association (Snyder 1991), and two by the National Association of School Nurses (Proctor 1990, 1993).

The standards within this document were originally approved by the National Association of School Nurses Board of Directors in June 1998 as the *Standards of Professional School Nursing Practice*. These have been reviewed by the American School Health Association, the National Association of State School Nurse Consultants, and the National Nursing Coalition for School Health. The standards serve as a definitive guide for role implementation, interpretation, and evaluation. They may be used separately or together with state nurse practice acts, scope of practice statements, and other relevant laws or statutes in determining the adequacy and competency of school nursing practice.

The scope statement describes the who, what, where, when, why, and how of the specialty. Extensive review and discussion by professional school nurses focused on answering these questions and resulted in this scope statement which was reviewed and approved by the Board of Directors of the National Association of School Nurses in 2000. The combination of the scope statement and standards provide a framework for the professional expectations of nurses who serve the students in our nation's schools and further define and clarify the role of nursing within schools and the school community.

SCOPE OF
PROFESSIONAL SCHOOL NURSING PRACTICE

Definitions and Distinguishing Characteristics

School nursing is a specialized practice of professional nursing that advances the well-being, academic success, and life-long achievement of students. School nursing takes place primarily within local education agencies serving school-age children. However, school nurses also provide services in alternative sites (e.g., juvenile justice centers, alternative treatment centers, preschools, and residential campuses) and within the larger surrounding community, at students' homes, vocational/occupational settings, environmental camps, field trips, school-sanctioned competitions, and sporting events.

The school nurse may be the only health care provider in the educational setting. Unlike other health care workers, such as occupational therapists, physical therapists, and school psychologists who have specific caseloads, the school nurse is responsible for all students in the school. School nurses are frequently called upon to delegate nursing care to teachers, school office staff, classroom assistants, and other unlicensed assistive personnel (UAP). School nurses must be fully aware of the applicable laws, regulations, and standards pertaining to delegation of nursing tasks to others. Some states may have laws or regulations in place prohibiting such delegation in the education setting.

Although health systems such as public health, hospitals, and private health care corporations may be the employer, school nurses are most commonly employed by local school districts or education systems. School nurses work in a variety of delivery models such as consultant, direct service delivery, and others. They work with individuals as well as populations, serving students from birth through age 21, or in some cases even older. School nurses, as active members of the interdisciplinary student services team, facilitate positive responses to normal development, promote health and safety, intervene with actual and potential health problems, provide case management services, and actively collaborate with others to build student and family capacity for adaptation, self-management, self-advocacy, and learning.

Historically, school nursing began in the early twentieth century as a result of efforts by public health nurses to combat high rates of school absenteeism due to communicable disease outbreaks among students (Smith and Mauer 2000). In today's world, communicable diseases are not the only health-related barriers to education. Some of the issues school nurses must address currently include child abuse/neglect; domestic and school violence; child and adolescent obesity; suicide; alcohol, tobacco, and other drug use; adolescent pregnancy and parenting; environmental health; mental health; lack of health insurance coverage; and more.

School nursing is the pivotal component in continuity of care through the coordination, planning, provision, and assessment of school health services. School nurses use the nursing process, as outlined in the accompanying Standards of Professional School Nursing Practice (originally published by NASN in 1998) , to implement strategies that promote student and staff health and safety. They develop team relationships within the school and with community health providers so that care is coordinated across settings to meet individual health needs and to avoid duplication of efforts and services.

The school nurse's primary role is to support student learning by acting as an advocate and liaison between the home, the school, and the medical community regarding concerns that are likely to affect a student's ability to learn (NASN 1999). The school nurse provides comprehensive services in all eight components of a coordinated school health program (Marx, Wooley, and Northrup 1998):

- Health services—Serves as the coordinator of the health services program, provides nursing care, and advocates for health rights.

- Health education—Provides appropriate health information that promotes informed health care decisions, promotes health, prevents disease, and enhances school performance.

- Environment—Identifies health and safety concerns in the school community and promotes a safe and nurturing school environment.

- Nutrition—Supports school food service programs and promotes the benefits of healthy eating patterns.

- Physical education/activity—Promotes healthy activities, physical education, and sports policies/practices that promote safety and good sportsmanship.

- Counseling/mental health—Provides health counseling, assesses mental health needs, provides interventions, refers students to appropriate school staff or community agencies, and provides follow-up once treatment is prescribed.

- Parent/community involvement—Promotes community participation in assuring a healthy school and serves as school liaison to a health advisory committee.

- Staff wellness—Provides health education and counseling, promotes healthy activities and environment for school staff.

Levels of Practice

Two levels of professional school nursing practice exist. Both the school nurse, who is a generalist, and the school nurse practitioner, who has advanced practice training, must hold current licensure as registered nurses in the state in which they practice. Additionally, school nurse practitioners must also hold current licensure as an advanced practice nurse in the state in which they practice, if such licensure exists in that state.

Because of the complexity of issues addressed by the school nurse, the National Association of School Nurses (NASN) recommends that the minimum educational preparation for a school nurse be a baccalaureate degree from an accredited college or university and school nurse certification (NASN 1996).

It is understood that there are school nurse generalists and school nurse practitioners who have not acquired these credentials. All school nurse generalists and school nurse practitioners are, however, encouraged to aspire to and achieve these qualifications.

School nurses, whether generalists or advanced practice nurses, utilize a public health focus in their practice. Health services are provided within the framework of primary, secondary, and tertiary prevention. Programs and health services are offered—with the goal of prevention—to individual students as well as to the entire school community.

Generalist

The school nurse is a registered professional nurse who has completed a formal course of study from a school of nursing. The school nurse functions to strengthen and facilitate students' educational outcomes. The school nurse provides preventive health, health assessment, and referral services to students. The actions of the school nurse may be directed toward individual students, family, school community, the larger surrounding community, aggregates within the school population, or the entire school population. The school nurse serves as the liaison between the school, community health care providers and the school-based or school-linked clinic.

A school nurse needs expertise in pediatric, community health, adult, and mental health nursing with strong health promotion, assessment, referral, communication, leadership, organization, and time management skills. Knowledge of health and education laws impacting children is essential, as are teaching strategies for the delivery of health education to students and staff.

The functions of the school nurse are to promote academic success and provide optimal nursing care to the entire school community. These functions include (ANA 1998):

- Assessment—Data collection.

- Diagnosis—Formulating nursing diagnosis based on data analysis.

- Outcome identification—Specifying appropriate and realistic expectations that are measurable.

- Planning—Developing a plan of care with interventions to attain the expected outcomes.

- Implementation—Providing interventions identified in the plan of care.

- Evaluation—Assessing progress toward attainment of the outcomes.

Advanced Practice

The school nurse practitioner is a registered professional nurse who has completed a formal course of study at a post-baccalaureate level. They have an expanded role beyond the scope of the school nurse generalist. School nurse practitioners provide primary health care to students registered to receive care in school-based and school-linked clinics or act as district employees to provide comprehensive health services to all students. Their practice builds on previous nursing knowledge and utilizes the nursing process (NASN 1995). They collaborate with school nurses, other health care professionals, and educators. School nurse practitioners provide health assessments and appropriate health counseling and treatment for students. These functions, which may include prescriptive authority for medications and treatments, are dependent on individual state laws and regulations.

Certification

School nurse generalists have the opportunity to demonstrate their knowledge of school nursing by acquiring certification in the nursing specialty of school nursing. The bachelor's degree is the minimum level of education required to sit for the national school nurse certification examination. Some state education agencies have a certification process for school nurses that is not a nursing specialty practice certification. Advanced practice school nurses must have a master's degree and/or hold national certification as a nurse practitioner or a clinical nurse specialist (NASN 1997).

Ethical Considerations

The degree to which the school environment supports nursing practice affects the delivery of nursing care. *Healthy People 2010* cites a recommended school nurse to student ratio of 1:750 in the national health objectives (USDHHS 2000). School nurses must be able to practice nursing in an educationally focused system and communicate clearly within both the health care and education arenas. They face unique policy, funding, and supervisory issues.

The school nurse practices in an environment that has changed dramatically since the early 20th century. The Individuals with Disabilities Act of 1997, section 504 of the Rehabilitation Act of 1973, and the Americans with Disabilities Act have contributed to removing barriers that in the past have hindered students' access to education. Education regulations heighten the complexity of decision making and practice (e.g., the Family Educational Rights and

Privacy Act [FERPA] of 1974 and subsequent amendments, respecting Do Not Resuscitate Orders in the School Setting).

School nurses are advocates for students, families, school staff, and the community. They facilitate positive responses to normal development, promote health and safety, and intervene with actual and potential health problems.

School nurses provide age-appropriate, culturally and ethnically sensitive care to students, families, the school community, and the larger surrounding community. They support active participation in health decisions. School nurses respect individual rights to be treated with dignity. School nurses understand the ethical and legal issues surrounding an individual's right to privacy and confidentiality. Regardless of race, gender, social or economic status, culture, age, sexual orientation, disability, or religion, the school nurse treats all members of the school community equally.

The school nurse maintains the highest level of competency by enhancing professional knowledge and skills and by collaborating with peers and other health professionals and community agencies, adhering to the Standards of Professional School Nursing Practice. School nurses participate in the profession's efforts to advance the standards of practice, expand the body of knowledge through nursing research, and improve conditions of employment.

Conclusions

School nurses continue to adapt their practice to an ever-changing world. New challenges continue to present, as do new tools to assist the school nurse in meeting those challenges. As technology advances, so does its use in the school nurse's practice. Technology is available not only as a classroom tool but also allows students with health impairments greater access to the education they are entitled to receive.

School nurses exist to support student success through health promotion and prevention at all levels (primary, secondary, and tertiary). On a primary level, the school nurse provides health information in classrooms and on an individual basis, refers students for appropriate immunizations, and promotes student and staff wellness. On a secondary level, school nurses facilitate vision, hearing, spinal, and other screening. The tertiary level of health promotion and prevention is evident in the school nurse's role in the school management of chronic health problems such as asthma, diabetes, cystic fibrosis, spina bifida, and others. This has not changed since the inception of school nursing. School nurses today and in the future will continue to anticipate the needs of their clients and adapt their practice to meet these changes.

STANDARDS OF
PROFESSIONAL SCHOOL NURSING PRACTICE

Background

Definition and Role of Standards

Standards are authoritative statements by which the nursing profession describes responsibilities for which its practitioners are accountable. Consequently, standards reflect the values and priorities of the profession. Standards provide direction for professional nursing practice and a framework for the evaluation of practice. Written in measurable terms, standards also define the nursing profession's accountability to the public and the client outcomes for which nurses are responsible (ANA 1998, p. 1).

Guidelines, as distinguished from standards, "describe a process of patient [client] care management which has the potential for improving the quality of clinical and consumer decision making. Guidelines are systematically developed statements based on available scientific evidence and expert opinion. Guidelines address the care of specific patient [client] populations or phenomena, whereas standards provide a broad framework for practice" (ANA 1998, p. 4).

Within school nursing, considerable professional literature is available that may be considered guidelines. Position statements and other publications of the National Association of School Nurses, the American School Health Association, the American Public Health Association's Public Health Nursing Section, the National Association of State School Nurse Consultants, the American Nurses' Association, and others, when specific to aspects of school nursing practice, may be regarded as guidelines.

Development of Standards

"A professional nursing organization has a responsibility to its membership and the public it serves to develop standards of practice" (ANA 1998, p. 1). This document sets forth standards of clinical practice for the specialty of school nursing and describes a competent level of professional performance common to all nurses engaged in the practice of school nursing.

Assumptions

1. The link between the work environment and the nurse's ability to deliver care and services is recognized, and employers must provide an environment supportive of nursing practice.

2. Nursing care is individualized to meet client needs and situations, including family goals and preferences. Given that one of the nurse's primary responsibilities is client health education, the school nurse provides clients with appropriate information to make informed decisions regarding their health care, including information that promotes health, prevents disease, and enhances school performance.

3. The school nurse works collaboratively to coordinate health and other services as needed to maximize the educational potential of the client. Collaboration involves partnerships with the family, other school professionals, and community health and social service providers and agencies.

Organizing Principles of the Standards of Professional School Nursing Practice

The Standards of Professional School Nursing Practice are on the parent document, *Standards of Clinical Nursing Practice* (ANA 1998). The parent document has two sections, "Standards of Care" and "Standards of Professional Performance." The Standards of Care are familiar to all nurses and constitute the nursing process. The Standards of Professional Performance constitute a framework for professional behavior. Consonant with the American Nurses Association's Social Policy Statement (ANA 1995), "the recipients of nursing care are individuals, groups, families, or communities . . . the individual recipient of nursing care can be referred to as patient, client, or person" (ANA 1998, p. 2). Throughout this document, client, when used, may refer to an individual, family, group, or community.

INTRODUCTION TO STANDARDS

The Standards of Care, composed of the six steps of the nursing process, describe a competent level of nursing care for all nurses, regardless of practice setting. "The nursing process encompasses all significant actions taken by nurses in providing care to all clients, and forms the foundation for clinical decision making" (ANA 1998, p. 3).

Standards of Care

- Standard I: Assessment

- Standard II: Diagnosis

- Standard III: Outcome Identification

- Standard IV: Planning

- Standard V: Implementation

- Standard VI: Evaluation

The original nursing process consisted of four steps: "Assessment," "Planning," "Implementation," and "Evaluation" (Yura and Walsh 1973). Due in large part to the work of Marjory Gordon (1976), Lynda Carpenito (1983), and others, "Diagnosis" was separated from "Assessment" and added as a logical outcome of "Assessment." In turn, "Outcome Identification" was identified as a product of "Diagnosis" because of the need to consider goals prior to any planning, as well as the emphasis on promoting and measuring outcomes of care (ANA 1991).

In addition to the nursing process and its prescriptive mandate for competent care, "several themes cut across all areas of nursing practice and reflect nursing responsibilities for all patients [clients]." These themes include:

- "providing age-appropriate, culturally, and ethnically sensitive care;

- maintaining a safe environment;

- educating patients [clients] about healthy practices and treatment modalities;

- assuring continuity of care;

- coordinating care across settings and among care givers;

- managing information; and

- communicating effectively." (ANA 1998, p. 3)

The themes are reflected throughout this document within criteria associated with the standards, although the language may differ somewhat. The themes are noted here because they (1) are fundamental to many of the standards, and (2) consistently and significantly influence contemporary school nursing practice.

Standards of Professional Performance

The Standards of Professional Performance describe a competent level of behavior in the professional role. "All nurses are expected to engage in professional role activities appropriate to their education and position. Ultimately, nurses are accountable to themselves, their patients [clients], and their peers for their professional activities" (ANA 1998, p. 3).

The Standards Task Force added three standards to the grouping, appearing below as the last three standards in the list. Two of the three additional standards (10 and 11) were taken from the *Standards of School Nursing Practice* (ANA 1983) while the third (9) was gleaned from NASN's standards implementation document (Proctor, Lordi, and Zaiger 1993).

- Standard I: Quality of Care
- Standard II: Performance Appraisal
- Standard III: Education
- Standard IV: Collegiality
- Standard V: Ethics
- Standard VI: Collaboration
- Standard VII: Research
- Standard VIII: Resource Utilization
- Standard IX: Communication
- Standard X: Program Management
- Standard XI: Health Education

Criteria

The criteria immediately following each standard statement are indicators or benchmarks of competent practice. The Standards of Professional School Nursing Practice include criteria that allow the standards to be measured. Standards generally remain stable over time, reflecting the philosophical values of the specialty. Criteria, however, must be revised to incorporate changes in practice and research and maintain consistency with current advances in scientific knowledge and clinical practice.

Because a document such as this cannot account for all possible developments in practice, modifiers such as "pertinent," "appropriate," and "realistic" may be used, which recognize differences in practice arenas, educational preparation, and scope of practice. Guidelines, documents, and local protocols and procedures, as well as state nurse practice acts, may provide additional direction if further interpretation is needed.

Summary

The Standards of Professional School Nursing Practice delineates the professional responsibilities of all school nurses engaged in clinical practice. The use of this and other documents could serve as a basis for:

- quality improvement systems;
- data bases;
- regulatory systems;
- health care reimbursement and financing methodologies;
- development and evaluation of nursing service delivery systems and organizational structures;
- certification activities;
- position descriptions and performance appraisals;
- agency policies, procedures, and protocols; and
- educational offerings.

Standards, as well as practice guidelines, must be evaluated on a regular basis. School nurses are invited to provide feedback to the Standards of Practice Task Force regarding the utility, effectiveness, and comprehensiveness of these standards.

STANDARDS OF CARE OF
PROFESSIONAL SCHOOL NURSING PRACTICE

Standard I. Assessment

The school nurse collects client data.

Measurement Criteria

1. Data collection involves the student, family, school staff, community, and other providers, as necessary.

2. The priority of data collection is determined by the nursing diagnosis and the client's immediate condition and/or needs.

3. Pertinent individual and aggregate data are collected, using appropriate assessment techniques, and reviewed in light of relevant supporting information.

4. Relevant data are documented in a retrievable form.

5. The data collection process is systematic, organized, and ongoing.

Standard II. Diagnosis

The school nurse analyzes the assessment data in determining nursing diagnoses.

Measurement Criteria

1. Nursing diagnoses, individual and aggregate, are derived from the evaluation of assessment data.

2. Nursing diagnoses, individual and aggregate, are validated with the student, family, school staff, community, and other providers, when appropriate.

3. Nursing diagnoses, individual and aggregate, are documented in a manner that facilitates the determination of expected outcomes and the plan of care/action.

Standard III. Outcome Identification

The school nurse identifies expected outcomes individualized to the client.

Measurement Criteria

1. Outcomes are derived from the nursing diagnoses.
2. Outcomes are mutually formulated with the student, family, school staff, community, and other providers, as appropriate.
3. Outcomes are culturally appropriate and realistic in relation to the client's present and potential capabilities.
4. Outcomes are obtained in relation to resources necessary and attainable.
5. Outcomes include a reasonable time line.
6. Outcomes provide direction for continuity of care and the plan of care/action.
7. Outcomes are documented as measurable goals.

Standard IV. Planning

The school nurse develops a plan of care/action that specifies interventions to attain expected outcomes.

Measurement Criteria

1. The plan is individualized to the student's diagnosis/nursing diagnosis.
2. A plan is a component of the individual program for students with special health care needs.
3. The plan is developed in compliance with local, state, and federal regulations, as needed.
4. The plan is collaboratively developed with the student, family, school staff, community, and other providers, as appropriate.

5. The plan reflects current standards of school nursing practice.

6. The plan provides for continuity of care and plan of action to be taken.

7. Priorities for care/action and time line for interventions are established.

8. The plan is documented in a retrievable form.

Standard V. Implementation

The school nurse implements the interventions identified in the plan of care/action.

Measurement Criteria

1. Interventions are consistent with the established plan of care/action.

2. Interventions are implemented in a safe, timely, and appropriate manner.

3. Interventions are documented in a retrievable form.

4. Interventions reflect current standards of school nursing practice.

Standard VI. Evaluation

The school nurse evaluates the client's progress toward attainment of outcomes.

Measurement Criteria

1. Evaluation is systematic, continuous, and criterion based.

2. The student, family, school staff, community, and other providers are involved in the evaluation process, as appropriate.

3. Ongoing assessment data, including incremental goal attainment in achieving the expected outcomes, are used to revise

diagnoses and outcomes and the plan of care/action, as needed.

4. Revisions in nursing diagnoses, outcomes, and the plan of care/action are documented in a retrievable form.

5. The client's responses to interventions are documented in a retrievable form.

6. The effectiveness of interventions is evaluated in relation to outcomes.

STANDARDS OF PROFESSIONAL PERFORMANCE OF PROFESSIONAL SCHOOL NURSING PRACTICE

Standard I. Quality of Care

The school nurse systematically evaluates the quality and effectiveness of school nursing practice.

Measurement Criteria

1. The school nurse participates in quality assurance activities as appropriate to that individual's position and practice environment. Such activities may include:

    *   identification of aspects of care necessary for quality monitoring;

    *   development of policies, procedures, and adoption of practice guidelines to improve quality of care;

    *   collection of data to monitor the quality and effectiveness of nursing care;

    *   formulation of recommendations to improve school nursing practice or client outcomes;

    *   implementation of activities to enhance the quality of nursing practice; and

    *   evaluation/research to test quality and effectiveness.

2. The school nurse uses the results of quality of care activities to initiate changes in school nursing practice, as appropriate.

3. The school nurse continuously strives to improve the quality and effectiveness of school health services.

Standard II. Performance Appraisal

The school nurse evaluates one's own nursing practice in relation to professional practice standards and relevant statutes, regulations, and policies.

Measurement Criteria

1. The school nurse participates in performance appraisal on a regular basis, identifying areas of strength and weakness, as well as ways to refine professional development.

2. The school nurse seeks and acts on constructive feedback regarding one's own practice.

3. The school nurse takes action to achieve goals identified during performance appraisal.

4. The school nurse initiates and participates in peer review, as appropriate.

5. The school nurse's practice reflects knowledge of current professional practice standards, education and health care laws and regulations, and school policies.

Standard III. Education

The school nurse acquires and maintains current knowledge and competency in school nursing practice.

Measurement Criteria

1. The school nurse acquires knowledge and skills appropriate to the specialty practice of school nursing on a regular and ongoing basis.

2. The school nurse consistently participates in continuing education activities related to current clinical knowledge and professional issues.

3. The school nurse seeks experience to maintain current clinical skills and competence.

Standard IV. Collegiality

The school nurse interacts with and contributes to the professional development of peers and school personnel as colleagues.

Measurement Criteria

1. The school nurse shares knowledge and skills with nursing and interdisciplinary colleagues.

2. The school nurse provides peers with constructive feedback regarding their practice.

3. The school nurse interacts with nursing and interdisciplinary colleagues to enhance professional practice and the health care of students.

4. The school nurse contributes to an environment that is conducive to clinical education of nursing students, other health care students, and other employees.

5. The school nurse contributes to a supportive and healthy work environment.

6. The school nurse participates in appropriate professional organizations in a membership and/or leadership capacity.

Standard V. Ethics

The school nurse's decisions and actions on behalf of clients are determined in an ethical manner.

Measurement Criteria

1. The school nurse's practice is guided by the Code for Nurses (ANA 1985) and Code of Ethics with Interpretative Statement for School Nurses (NASN 1999), and appropriate state nurse practice acts.

2. The school nurse maintains client confidentiality within legal, regulatory, and ethical parameters of health and education.

3. The school nurse delivers care in a nonjudgmental and nondiscriminatory manner that is sensitive to student diversity in the school community.

4. The school nurse delivers care in a manner that promotes and preserves student and family autonomy, dignity, and rights.

5. The school nurse seeks available resources to formulate ethical decisions.

6. The school nurse acts as a client advocate.

Standard VI. Collaboration

The school nurse collaborates with the student, family, school staff, community, and other providers in providing student care.

Measurement Criteria

1. The school nurse communicates verbally and in writing with the student, family, school staff, community, and other providers regarding client care and nursing's role in the provision of care.

2. The school nurse collaborates with the student, family, school staff, community, and other providers in the formulation of overall goals, time lines, the plan of care, and decisions related to care and the delivery of services.

3. The school nurse assists individual students in developing appropriate skills to advocate for themselves based on age and developmental level.

4. The school nurse consults with and utilizes the expertise of other providers for client care, as needed.

5. The school nurse makes referrals, including provisions for continuity of care, as needed.

Standard VII. Research

The school nurse promotes use of research findings in school nursing practice.

Measurement Criteria

1. The school nurse utilizes available research in developing the health programs and individual client plans of care and interventions.

2. The school nurse participates in research activities as appropriate to the nurse's education, position, and practice environment. Such activities may include:

   • identifying clinical problems suitable for nursing research;

   • participating in data collection;

   • participating in a unit, organization, or community research committee or program;

   • interpreting research findings with others;

   • conducting research;

   • critiquing research for application to practice; and

   • using research findings in the development of policies and procedures for client care and program development.

3. The school nurse contributes to the nursing literature when possible.

Standard VIII. Resource Utilization

The school nurse considers factors related to safety, effectiveness, and cost when planning and delivering care.

Measurement Criteria

1. The school nurse evaluates factors related to safety, effectiveness, availability, and cost when choosing between two or more practice options that would result in the same expected client or program outcomes.

2. The school nurse assists the student, family, school staff, and community in identifying and securing appropriate and available services and resources to address health-related needs.

3. The school nurse assigns or delegates tasks as defined by the state nurse practice acts and according to the knowledge and skills of the designated care giver.

4. If the school nurse assigns or delegates tasks, it is based on the needs and condition of the client and potential for harm, the stability of the client's condition, the complexity of the task, and the predictability of the outcome.

5. The school nurse assists the student, family, school staff, and community in becoming informed consumers about the cost, risks, and benefits of health promotions, health education, school health services, and individualized health interventions for students.

Standard IX. Communication

The school nurse uses effective written, verbal, and nonverbal communication skills.

Measurement Criteria

1. The school nurse communicates effectively with the student, family, school staff, community, and other providers regarding student care and the role of the school nurse in the provision of care.

2. The school nurse employs counseling techniques and crisis intervention strategies for individuals and groups.

3. The school nurse utilizes communication as a positive strategy to achieve nursing goals.

4. The school nurse demonstrates knowledge of the philosophy and mission of the school district, the kind and nature of its curricular and extracurricular activities, and its programs and special services.

5. The school nurse demonstrates knowledge of the roles of other school professionals and adjunct personnel, and coordinates roles and responsibilities of the adjunct school health personnel within the school team.

Note: The language of this Standard Statement and all measurement criteria 2 through 5 are taken or adapted from *School Nursing Practice: Roles and Standards* (Proctor, Lordi, and Zaiger 1993).

Standard X. Program Management

The school nurse manages school health services.

Measurement Criteria

1. The school nurse manages school health services as appropriate to the nurse's education, position, and practice environment.

2. The school nurse conducts school health needs assessments to identify current health problems and identify the need for new programs.

3. The school nurse develops and implements needed health programs using a program planning process.

4. The school nurse demonstrates knowledge of existing school health programs and current health trends that may impact client care, the sources of funds for each, school policy related to each, and local, state, and federal law governing each.

5. The school nurse develops and implements health policies and procedures in collaboration with school administration, board of health, and the board of education.

6. The school nurse evaluates ongoing health programs for outcomes and quality of care and communicates findings to administrators and the board of education.

7. The school nurse orients, provides training, documents competency, supervises, and evaluates health assistants, aides, and UAPs (Unlicensed Assistive Personnel), as appropriate to the school setting.

8. The school nurse uses the results of school health/environmental needs assessment, analysis of evaluation data, and quality of care activities to initiate changes throughout the health care delivery system, as appropriate.

9. The school nurse participates in environmental safety and health activities (e.g., indoor air quality, injury surveillance, and prevention).

10. The school nurse adopts and utilizes available technology, as appropriate to the work setting.

    Note: The language of this Standard Statement and all measurement criteria 2 through 7 are taken or adapted from *School Nursing Practice: Roles and Standards* (Proctor, Lordi, and Zaiger 1993).

Standard XI. Health Education

The school nurse assists students, families, the school staff, and community to achieve optimal levels of wellness through appropriately designed and delivered health education.

Measurement Criteria

1. The school nurse participates in the assessment of needs for health education and health instruction for the school community.

2. The school nurse provides formal health instruction within the classroom based on sound learning theory, as appropriate to student developmental levels.

3. The school nurse provides individual and group health teaching and counseling for and with clients.

4. The school nurse participates in the design and development of health curricula.

5. The school nurse participates in the evaluation of health curricula, health instructional materials, and other health education activities.

6. The school nurse acts as a resource person to school staff regarding health education and health education materials.

7. The school nurse furthers the application of health promotion principles within all areas of school life (e.g., food service, custodial, etc.).

8. The school nurse promotes self-care and safety through the education of staff regarding their own health and that of their students.

   Note: The language of this Standard Statement and all measurement criteria are taken or adapted from *School Nursing Practice: Roles and Standards* (Proctor, Lordi, and Zaiger 1993).

GLOSSARY

Assessment—The first step of the nursing process, assessment is the collection and documentation of data/information about or from individuals, students, families, health care providers, organizations, or communities in a systematic, continuous manner, using appropriate techniques (ANA 1998).

Client—A collective term, which may refer to individuals, families, groups, or communities who are the recipients of nursing care (ANA 1995).

Diagnosis—The second step of the nursing process, diagnosis is the analysis of the assessment data to arrive at a conclusion(s) that can be validated by others, is documented, and facilitates the development of outcomes and a plan of care (ANA 1998).

Evaluation—The sixth and final step of the nursing process, evaluation is a systematic and ongoing appraisal of client responses to interventions and to the effectiveness of interventions in relation to outcomes. Evaluative data are documented and used to revise assessments, diagnoses, outcomes, plans, and interventions (ANA 1998).

Implementation—The fifth step of the nursing process, implementation is the execution of the interventions prescribed in a safe, appropriate manner. Interventions are always documented (ANA 1998).

Outcome identification—The third and newest step of the nursing process, outcome identification is the specification of measurable, appropriate, mutually formulated, attainable, and timely goals that are derived from the diagnosis(es), are documented, and provide for continuity of care (ANA 1998).

Plan of care—A comprehensive outline of care to be delivered to attain expected outcomes (ANA 1998). Examples may include Individualized Health Plan, Individualized Education Plan, 504 plans, and others.

Planning—The fourth step of the nursing process, planning is a prescription of interventions designed to attain outcomes unique to the client which provide for continuity of care, are documented, and are conjointly created, when appropriate (ANA 1998).

School nursing—School nursing is a specialized practice of professional nursing that advances the well-being, academic success, and life-long achievement of students. To that end, school nurses facilitate positive student responses to normal development; promote health and safety; intervene with actual and potential health problems; provide case management services; and actively collaborate with others to build student and family capacity for adaptation, self management, self advocacy, and learning.

Standards—Standards are authoritative statements enunciated and promulgated by the profession by which the quality of practice, service, or education can be judged (ANA 1998).

REFERENCES

The following references apply to both the Scope of Professional School Nursing Practice and the Standards of Professional School Nursing Practice.

American Nurses Association (ANA). 1983. *Standards of School Nursing Practice.* Kansas City, MO: American Nurses Association.

———. 1985. *Code for Nurses with Interpretive Statements.* Kansas City, MO: American Nurses Publishing.

———. 1991. *Standards of Clinical Nursing Practice.* Kansas City, MO: American Nurses Publishing.

———. 1995. *Nursing's Social Policy Statement.* Washington, DC: American Nurses Publishing.

———. 1998. *Standards of Clinical Nursing Practice.* 2d ed. Washington, DC: American Nurses Publishing.

Carpenito, L. J. 1983. *Nursing Diagnosis: Application to Clinical Practice.* Philadelphia: Lippincott.

Gordon, M. 1976. Nursing diagnosis and the diagnostic process. *Journal of the New York State Nurses Association* 76:1276–1300.

Marx, E., Wooley, S., and Northrup, D., eds. 1998. *Health Is Academic: a Guide to Coordinated School Health Programs.* New York: Teacher's College Press.

National Association of School Nurses (NASN). 1988. *Philosophy of School Health Services and School Nursing.* Scarborough, ME: National Association of School Nurses.

———. 1995. *Position Statement, the School Nurse Practitioner.* Scarborough, ME: National Association of School Nurses.

————. 1996. *Position Statement, Professional School Nurse Roles and Responsibilities: Education, Certification, and Licensure.* Scarborough, ME: National Association of School Nurses.

————. 1997. *Position Statement, the Advance Practice School Nurse.* Scarborough, ME: National Association of School Nurses.

————. 1998. *Standards of Professional School Nursing Practice.* Scarborough, ME: National Association of School Nurses.

————. 1999. *Code of Ethics with Interpretive Statements for School Nurses.* Scarborough, ME: National Association of School Nurses.

————. 1999. *The Role of the School Nurse.* [Brochure]. Scarborough, ME: National Association of School Nurses.

Proctor, S. T. 1990. *Guidelines for a Model School Nurse Services Program.* Scarborough, ME: National Association of School Nurses.

Proctor, S. T., with Lordi, S. L., and Zaiger, D. S. 1993. *School Nursing Practice: Roles and Standards.* Scarborough, ME: National Association of School Nurses.

Smith, C. M., and Mauer, F. A., eds. 2000. *Community Health Nursing: Theory and Practice.* 2d ed. Philadelphia: Saunders.

Snyder, A. A., ed. 1991. *Implementation Guide for the Standards of School Nursing Practice.* Kent, OH: American School Health Association.

U.S. Department of Health and Human Services (USDHHS). 2000. *Healthy People 2010: Health Objectives for the Nation.* Washington, D.C.: U.S. Department of Health and Human Services.

Yura, H., and Walsh, M. B. 1973. *The Nursing Process: Assessing, Planning, Implementing, Evaluating.* 2d. ed. New York: Appleton-Century-Crofts.

ACKNOWLEDGMENTS

The National Association of School Nurses gratefully acknowledges the careful and useful critique of draft manuscripts by the following reviewers:

American Nurses Association

American Public Health Association

American School Health Association

National Association of Pediatric Nurse Associates and Practitioners

National Association of State School Nurse Consultants

National Center for School Health Nursing

Standards of Practice Task Force

Charla Dunham, RN, BSN, MEd, Chair; Standards/Practice Issues Committee
National Association of School Nurses, Inc.

Nancy Birchmeier, RN, BSN, NCSN; Standards/Practice Issues Committee
National Association of School Nurses, Inc.

Linda Edwards, RN, DrPH; Organizational Representative
American Public Health Association, Public Health Nursing Section

Beverly Farquhar, RN, BS, NCSN; Executive Director
National Association of School Nurses, Inc.

Tona Leiker, RN, MN; Organizational Representative
American Nurses Association

Doris Luckenbill, RN, MS, CRNP; President
National Association of School Nurses, Inc.

Judith A. Maire, RN, MN; Organizational Representative
National Association of State School Nurse Consultants

Susan Proctor, RN, DNS; Author, *School Nursing Practice:*
Roles and Standards
National Association of School Nurses, Inc.

Genie Wessel, RN, MS, FASHA; Organizational Representative
American School Health Association

Linda Wolfe, RN, BSN, MEd, NCSN; Past Chair,
Standards/Practice Issues Committee
National Association of School Nurses, Inc.

Other Reviewers

Elaine Brainerd, RN, MA, NCSN; Director, National Center for
School Health Nursing American Nurses Association/Foundation

Leslie Cooper, RN, MSN, CS, FNP; Standards/Practice Issues
Committee, Board Member (Kentucky), National Association of
School Nurses, Inc.

Donna Mazyck, RN, BSN, NCSN; Standards/Practice Issues
Committee, Board Member (Maryland), National Association of
School Nurses, Inc.

Donna Zaiger, RN, BSN, NCSN; Past President
National Association of School Nurses, Inc.

Library of Congress Cataloging-in-Publication Data

National Association of School Nurses (U.S.)
   Scope and standards of professional school nursing practice /
National Association of School Nurses, Inc. [and] American Nurses
Association.
      p. ; cm.
   Includes bibliographical references.
   ISBN 1-55810-163-2 (alk. paper)
   1. School nursing—Standards—United States. 2. School nursing—
Study and teaching—United States. I. American Nurses' Association.
II. Title.
   [DNLM: 1. School Nursing—standards—United States. 2. School
Nursing—education—United States. WY 113 N277s 2001]
RT85.5 .N385 2001
371.7'12'0973—dc21

2001022682

Published by
American Nurses Publishing
600 Maryland Avenue, SW
Suite 100 West
Washington, D.C. 20024-2571

ISBN 1-55810-163-2

SHNP21   3M   06/01

INDEX

A year in brackets [2001] indicates an entry from *Scope and Standards of Professional School Nursing Practice* (2001), reproduced in Appendix A.

A
Administration, 6, 41
Advanced practice school nursing, 4
  [2001] 52, 53–54
  assessment, 9–10
  collaboration, 31
  collegiality, 29
  consultation, 20
  coordination of care, 17
  defined, 6
  [2001] 53
  diagnosis, 11
  education, 27
  ethics, 32
  evaluation, 22–23
  health teaching and health
    promotion, 18–19
  implementation, 16–21
  leadership, 38–39
  outcomes identification, 12–13
  planning, 14–15
  prescriptive authority and treatment,
    21
  professional practice evaluation, 28
  program management, 40
  quality of practice, 25–26
  research, 34
  resource utilization, 36
  roles, 6
  See also Generalist school nursing;
    Role specialty school nursing;
    School nursing
Advocacy for clients and families, 2, 3,
  7
  [2001] 50, 51, 55
  collaboration and, [2001] 70
  ethics and, 5, 32

Age-appropriate care. *See* Cultural
  competence
American Nurses Association (ANA), *vii*
  [2001] 57
  Code of Ethics with Interpretive
    Statements, 7, 32
  Code for Nurses with Interpretive
    Statements, [2001] 69
  Nursing: Scope and Standards of
    Practice, *vii*, *viii*
  Nursing's Social Policy Statement, 7
    [2001] 58
  Standards of Clinical Nursing Practice,
    [2001] 48, 58
American Public Health Association,
  [2001] 57
American School Health Association, *vii*
  [2001] 48, 57
Americans with Disabilities Act (1990), 7
  [2001] 54
Analysis. *See* Critical thinking, analysis,
  and synthesis
Assessment, *ix*, 3, 5
  [2001] 51, 53, 54, 59
  defined, [2001] 76
  diagnosis and, 11
  [2001] 63
  evaluation and, 22
  [2001] 65
  health education and, [2001] 74
  health teaching and health promotion,
    18
  planning and, 14
  program management and, 40
  [2001] 73, 74
  standard of practice, *xii*, 9–10
  [2001] 63

Critical thinking, analysis, and
synthesis, 4
assessment and, 9, 10
collaboration and, 31
consultation and, 20
coordination of care and, 17
diagnosis and, 11
evaluation and, 22, 23
[2001] 65
health teaching and health
promotion, 19
nursing process and, *ix*,
program management and, 40
[2001] 74
quality of practice and, 25, 26
research and, 34, 35
[2001] 71
resource utilization and, 36
Cultural competence, *ix*
[2001] 55, 60
ethics and, 7, 32
[2001] 70
health teaching and health promotion,
18, 19
outcomes identification and, 12
[2001] 64
planning and, 14, 15
professional practice evaluation and,
28

D
Data collection, [2001] 53, 60
assessment and, 5, 9
[2001] 63
quality of care and, [2001] 67
quality of practice and, 25
research and, 34
[2001] 71
Databases, *ix*, *x*
[2001] 62
Decision-making
[2001] 51, 54, 55, 57, 59
collaboration and, 31
[2001] 70
consultation and, 20
ethics and, 7, 33
leadership and, 39

planning and, 15
professional practice evaluation and,
28
research and, 34
Diagnosis, *ix*, 3, 5
[2001] 53, 59
assessment and, 9, 10
[2001] 63
defined, [2001] 76
evaluation and, 22
[2001] 65
implementation and, 16
outcomes identification and, [2001] 64
planning and, 14
[2001] 64
prescriptive authority and treatment,
21
standard of practice, *xii*, 11
[2001] 63
Documentation, *ix*, 8
assessment and, 10
[2001] 63
collaboration and, 31
coordination of care and, 17
diagnosis and, 11
[2001] 63
education and, 27
evaluation and, 22, 23
[2001] 66
implementation and, 16
[2001] 65
outcomes identification and, 12
[2001] 64
planning and, [2001] 65
program management and, 40
[2001] 73
quality of practice and, 25
Do Not Resuscitate orders, 7
[2001] 55

E
Economic issues. *See* Cost control
Education of clients and families, *ix*, 2, 3,
4, 5
[2001] 51, 52, 55, 57, 60, 74–75
coordination of care and, 17
resource utilization and, 36

Generalist school nursing (*continued*)
education, 27
ethics, 32
evaluation, 22
health teaching and health
   promotion, 18
implementation, 16–20
leadership, 38–39
outcomes identification, 12–13
planning, 14
professional practice evaluation, 28
program management, 40
quality of practice, 25–26
research, 34
resource utilization, 36
roles, 5–6
   [2001] 53
See also Advanced school nursing;
   Role specialty school nursing;
   School nursing
Guidelines, *x*
   [2001] 57, 62
leadership and, 39
outcomes identification and, 13
professional practice evaluation and,
   28
quality of care and, [2001] 67
quality of practice and, 26

H
Health education
   standard of professional performance,
   [2001] 74–75
Health Information Portability and
   Accessibility Act (HIPAA, 1996), 7
Health teaching and health promotion,
   3, 4–5
   [2001] 50, 51, 52, 53, 54, 55, 56
planning and, 14
standard of practice, *xii*, 18–19
resource utilization and, 36
   [2001] 72
Healthcare policy, *x*, 5
   [2001] 54, 62
evaluation and, 22, 23
leadership and, 39

program management and, 40
   [2001] 73
quality of care and, [2001] 67
quality of practice and, 26
research and, 34
   [2001] 71
Healthcare providers
   [2001] 54, 55, 60
assessment and, 9
   [2001] 63
collaboration and, 1, 31
   [2001] 70
communication and, [2001] 72
diagnosis and, 11
   [2001] 63
ethics and, 7
evaluation and, 22
   [2001] 65
leadership and, 38, 39
outcomes identification and, 12
   [2001] 64
planning and, [2001] 64
professional practice evaluation and,
   28
See also Collaboration; Interdisciplinary health care; Referrals
Healthcare team. *See* Collaboration;
   Interdisciplinary health care
Healthy People 2010, 7
   [2001] 54
Holistic practice, 9
Human resources. *See* Professional
   development

I
Implementation, *ix*, 3, 5
   [2001] 53, 59
defined, [2001] 76
evaluation and, 22
program management and, [2001] 73
standard of practice, *xii*, 16–21
   [2001] 65
Individualized education plan (IEP), 41
   [2001] 76
Individualized healthcare plan (IHP), 41
   [2001] 76

Individuals with Disabilities Act (1997), 7
[2001] 54
Information. *See* Data collection
Insurance reimbursement, *x*
[2001] 62
Interdisciplinary health care, 2
  collaboration and, 31
  collegiality and, 29, 30
  [2001] 69
  coordination of care and, 17
  ethics and, 33
  leadership and, 39
  planning and, 15
  quality of practice and, 26
  resource utilization and, 36
  See also Collaboration; Healthcare providers
Internet, 19
Interventions, 1, 3
  [2001] 52, 55
  communication and, [2001] 72
  evaluation and, [2001] 66
  implementation and, 16
  [2001] 65
  planning and, 14
  [2001] 64, 65
  prescriptive authority and treatment, 21
  research and, [2001] 71
  resource utilization and, 36, 37
  [2001] 72

L

Laws, statutes, and regulations, *viii*, *x*, 1, 5
  [2001] 48, 50, 54, 55, 62
  ethics and, 7, 32
  [2001] 69
  evaluation and, 22
  leadership and, 38
  planning and, 14
  [2001] 64
  performance appraisal and, [2001] 68
  prescriptive authority and treatment, 21

professional practice evaluation and, 28
program management and, 40
  [2001] 73
resource utilization and, 36
  [2001] 72
  See also Ethics
Leadership, 4, 5, 41
  [2001] 53, 54
  collegiality and, 29
  [2001] 69
  coordination of care and, 17
  program management and, 40
  [2001] 73
  standard of professional performance, *xiii*, 38–39
Legal issues. *See* Laws, statutes, and regulations
Licensing. *See* Certification and credentialing

M

Measurement criteria. *See* Criteria
Mentoring
  collegiality and, 29, 30
  leadership and, 38
Multidisciplinary healthcare. *See* Interdisciplinary health care

N

National Association of School Nurse Consultants, [2001] 48, 57
National Association of School Nurses (NASN), *vii*, *viii*, *x*, 4
  [2001] 48, 49, 52, 57
National Board for Certification of School Nurses, 4
National Nursing Coalition for School Health, [2001] 48
Nurse Practitioner (NP), 6
  [2001] 52, 53
Nursing care standards. *See* Standards of care
Nursing process, *ix*, 2, 5
  [2001] 51, 54, 58, 59–60, 76, 77
  quality of practice and, 25
  See also Standards of Practice

Nursing standards. *See* Standards of
    practice; Standards of
    professional performance

O
Outcomes, 1, 5
    collaboration and, 31
    diagnosis and, 11
        [2001] 63
    ethics and, 32, 33
    evaluation and, 22
        [2001] 65–66
    leadership and, 39
    planning and, 14
        [2001] 64
    program management and, 40
        [2001] 73
    quality of care and, [2001] 67
    quality of practice and, 25
    resource utilization and, 36, 37
        [2001] 72
    See also Evaluation; Outcomes
        identification
Outcomes identification, *ix*, 3, 5
    [2001] 53, 59
    defined, [2001] 76
    standard of practice, *xii*, 12–13
        [2001] 64
    See also Outcomes

P
Parents. *See* Family
Patient. *See* Client
Performance appraisal, [2001] 62
    standard of professional performance,
        [2001] 68
Pharmacologic agents. *See* Prescriptive
    authority
Plan of care (defined), [2001] 76
Planning, *ix*, 3, 5
    [2001] 51, 53, 59
    collaboration and, 31
        [2001] 70
    consultation and, 20
    coordination of care and, 17
    defined, 41
        [2001] 77

diagnosis and, 11
    [2001] 63
evaluation and, 22
    [2001] 66
implementation and, 16
    [2001] 65
leadership and, 38
outcomes identification and, 12
    [2001] 64
program management and, 40
    [2001] 73
research and, [2001] 71
resource utilization and, 36
standard of practice, *xii*, 14–15
    [2001] 64–65
Policy. *See* Healthcare policy
Practice environment, *ix*
    [2001] 51, 55, 57
    collegiality and, 29
        [2001] 69
    coordination of care and, 17
    ethics and, 7, 8
    leadership and, 38
    outcomes identification and, 12
    planning and, 14
    program management and, 40
        [2001] 73, 74
    quality of care and, [2001] 67
    quality of practice and, 26
    research and, [2001] 71
    resource utilization and, 36
Practice settings, 1–2, 8
    [2001] 50, 53
Preceptors. *See* Mentoring
Prescriptive authority and treatment
    [2001] 54
    standard of practice, *xii*, 21
Privacy. *See* Confidentiality
Process. *See* Nursing process
Professional development, 4
    [2001] 55
    collegiality and, 29
    education and, 27
        [2001] 68
    ethics and, 7
    leadership and, 38
    performance appraisal and, [2001] 68

professional practice evaluation and, 28
See also Education; Leadership
Professional organizations, 38
collegiality and, [2001] 69
Professional performance. *See* Standards
of professional performance
Professional practice evaluation, *x*
collegiality and, 29
health teaching and health
promotion, 18
standard of professional
performance, *xiii*, 28
Program management
standard of professional
performance, *xiii*, 40
[2001] 73–74

Q
Quality improvement, *x*
[2001] 62
planning and, 15
Quality of care, [2001]
program management and, [2001]
73, 74
standard of professional performance,
[2001] 67
Quality of practice
ethics and, 8
leadership and, 38, 39
program management and, 40
resource utilization and, 36
standard of professional
performance, *xiii*, 25–26

R
Recipient of care. *See* Client
Referrals, 3, 5
[2001] 52, 53, 55
collaboration and, 31
[2001] 70
prescriptive authority and treatment,
21
See also Coordination of care
Regulatory issues. *See* Laws, statutes,
and regulations
Reimbursement, *x*
[2001] 62

Research, 6
[2001] 55
collaboration and, 31
education and, 27
ethics and, 8
planning and, 14
program management and, 40
quality of care and, [2001] 67
quality of practice and, 26
standard of professional
performance, *xiii*, 34–35
[2001] 71
See also Evidence-based practice
Resource utilization, *ix*, 5
[2001] 53
ethics and, 32
[2001] 70
health teaching and health
promotion, 19
outcomes identification and, [2001]
64
program management and, 40
[2001] 74
standard of professional
performance, *xiii*, 36–37
[2001] 71–72
Risk assessment
ethics and, 32, 33
health teaching and health promotion,
19
leadership and, 38
outcomes identification and, 12
prescriptive authority and treatment,
21
resource utilization and, 37
[2001] 72
Role specialty school nursing
assessment, 9–10
collaboration, 31
collegiality, 29–30
consultation, 20
coordination of care, 17
defined, 6, 41
diagnosis, 11
education, 27
ethics, 32–33
evaluation, 22–23

collaboration and, 31
[2001] 70
communication and, [2001] 72, 73
diagnosis and, 11
[2001] 63
evaluation and, [2001] 65
health education and, [2001] 74, 75
health teaching and health
promotion, 18
leadership and, 38
outcomes identification and, 12
[2001] 64
planning and, [2001] 64
resource utilization and, [2001] 72
Scientific findings. *See* Evidence-based
practice; Research
*Scope and Standards for Nurse
Administrators*, 6
*Scope and Standards of Professional
School Nursing Practice*, *x*, 45–82
Scope of practice, *vii*, *ix*, 1–8
[2001] 48–49, 50–56
advanced level, 6
[2001] 53–54
generalist level, 5–6
[2001] 53
role specialty, 6
Section 504 (Rehabilitation Act, 1973),
7, 41
[2001] 54, 76
Self-care and self-management, [2001]
50
ethics and, 32
health education and, [2001] 75
health teaching and health
promotion, 18
Settings. *See* Practice settings
Significant others. *See* Family
Standard (defined), [2001] 57, 77
Standards of care, [2001] 59–66
history, *vii*, *viii*
See also Standards of practice
Standards of practice, *ix*, *xii*, 9–23
assessment, 9–10
consultation, 20
coordination of care, 17

diagnosis, 11
evaluation, 22–23
health teaching and health promotion,
18–19
implementation, 16–21
organizing principles, [2001] 58
outcomes identification, 12–13
planning, 14–15
prescriptive authority and treatment,
21
Standards of professional performance,
ix, *xiii*, 25–40
[2001] 60
collaboration, 31
collegiality, 29–30
education, 27
ethics, 32–33
leadership, 38–39
professional practice evaluation, 28
quality of practice, 25–26
research, 34–35
resource utilization, 36–37
Synthesis. *See* Critical thinking, analysis,
and synthesis

T
Teaching. *See* Education; Health
teaching and health promotion
Teams and teamwork. *See*
Interdisciplinary health care
Terminology, 41
[2001] 76–77
diagnosis and, 11
implementation and, 16
outcomes identification and, 12
planning and, 14
Trends in school nursing, 8
[2001] 51, 54–55

U
Unlicensed assistive personnel (UAP),
1, 38, 40
[2001] 50, 73

W
Wald, Lillian, 2